MICROSCOPY HANDBOOKS 28

CW00922852

Biological Microtechnique

Royal Microscopical Society MICROSCOPY HANDBOOKS

01 An Introduction to the Optical Microscope (2nd Edn)
03 Specimen Preparation for Transmission Electron Microscopy of Materials
04 Histochemical Protein Staining Methods
05 X-Ray Microanalysis in Electron Microscopy for Biologists
06 Lipid Histochemistry
08 Maintaining and Monitoring the Transmission Electron Microscope
09 Qualitative Polarized Light Microscopy
11 An Introduction to Immunocytochemistry (2nd Edn)
12 Introduction to Scanning Acoustic Microscopy
15 Dictionary of Light Microscopy
16 Light Element Analysis in the Transmission Electron Microscope
17 Colloidal Gold: a New Perspective for Cytochemical Marking
18 Autoradiography: a Comprehensive Overview
19 Introduction to Crystallography (2nd Edn)
20 The Operation of Transmission and Scanning Electron Microscopes
21 Cryopreparation of Thin Biological Specimens for Electron Microscopy
22 An Introduction to Surface Analysis by Electron Spectroscopy
23 Basic Measurement Techniques for Light Microscopy
24 The Preparation of Thin Sections of Rocks, Minerals and Ceramics
25 The Role of Microscopy in Semiconductor Failure Analysis
26 Enzyme Histochemistry
27 *In Situ* Hybridization: a Practical Guide
28 Biological Microtechnique

Biological Microtechnique

J.B. Sanderson
Sir William Dunn School of Pathology,
South Parks Road, Oxford OX1 3RE, UK

In association with the Royal Microscopical Society

© BIOS Scientific Publishers Limited, 1994

First published in the United Kingdom 1994 by
BIOS Scientific Publishers Limited,
St Thomas House, Becket Street, Oxford, OX1 1SJ
Tel: 0865 726286 Fax: 0865 246823

Transferred to Digital Printing 2005

A CIP catalogue for this book is available from the British Library.

ISBN 1 872748 42 2

Typeset by AMA Graphics Ltd, Preston, UK

Preface

Although there is now a general trend towards molecular biochemistry in current biological research and clinical practice, there is nevertheless still a requirement to produce good microscopical preparations. However good the microscope, it cannot enhance poorly prepared specimens, which inevitably lead to unreliable results. With this in mind, *Biological Microtechnique* presents the reader with the newest and also the well-proven classical methods of slide making. A well-prepared specimen not only displays information effectively, but is in itself an achievement and a joy to make. At first sight, preparing a standard thin section appears straightforward, and is the technique most often used in histology laboratories; but there are other little-used techniques which can equally well inform microscopists and answer their questions. Furthermore, the professional reseacher can learn much from the techniques employed by skilled amateurs, who often produce far superior preparations from the more limited means at their disposal. While much of the information is directed towards the professional researcher, I have tried to bear the requirements of the amateur microscopist in mind. There is, for example, information on older microtomes, on hand-sharpening microtome knives, and references to the older literature and techniques more suited to the individual working without the facilities of a modern research institute.

This book gives a general introduction to biological microtechnique for the light microscope, for students, postgraduate workers and technicians who are new to microscopy. Most texts in this field are either out of print, or else concentrate upon producing and examining thin sections. This book has been divided chapter by chapter into the steps of preparation: fixing, embedding, microtomy or otherwise, and mounting the final preparation. Because of the present dearth of comprehensive texts on biological microtechnique for the light microscope, this handbook does not cover preparation techniques for electron microscopy, but references are given to complementary texts in this field.

Histology and microscopy are often, unfortunately, taught in isolation to students. This book is intended to present a basic introduction to biological microtechnique, and supplements the other titles on microscopy in the RMS Handbook series. It is not a handbook covering every commonly used protocol or staining method. Those that are selected have been chosen because they demonstrate general principles and materials used in preparing microscope slides. For example, many empirical methods for haematoxylin have been published and are readily available. A rational formula, Haematal 8, which is both simple and reliable to use is published here for this reason. An understanding of how techniques work leads to controlled manipulation and better interpretation and diagnosis.

A practical work on biological microtechnique has not been published for 20 years, yet significant advances have been made in biological specimen preparation. The resurgence of interest in light microscopical (particularly confocal) techniques, which have not been superseded by the electron microscope, and indeed complement it to a greater extent than hitherto, and the use of newer resin media for embedding in addition to wax, mean this book will appeal to students, undergraduates, technicians and research fellows in whose work microscopy plays a large part, or who wish to extend their repertoire of techniques. I have assumed that they will have recourse to academic libraries, and have included extensive references throughout. These are intended to introduce the reader to the basis of each technique and point to similar work. Although microtechnique is largely a conservative art, the demands of modern biological research have brought corresponding improvements, particularly in preserving the structural and functional elements of cells and tissues during fixation and embedding. Similar advances have been made in the automated instrumentation available. Where possible, modern equipment has been illustrated within the space available, but readers are advised to consult manufacturers' and suppliers' catalogues.

Notes have been included in the appendix to supplement the safety caveat published in all the Society's handbooks, and a table of selected refractive indices has been included. Since the refractive index of mountants and immersion media can readily change, they have been given to two decimal places only, whereas those of solvents have been given to three places. I have tried throughout to explain the reasons why operations are carried out in the way described, particularly in the chapter on microtomy. My own experience, from a technical viewpoint, is that this approach gives a better understanding of why a particular technique works and helps to develop a critical feedback for the microtomist. It is hoped that this will lead to better work and increased confidence. In this way, I hope that those who read this book will come to a firmer and greater understanding of biological microtechnique, which cannot be learnt and ultimately enjoyed except by practice.

My own professional training has been as a histologist and microscopist. As a member of the active amateur learned societies I have been indebted to many friends for what they have taught me. I would welcome, therefore, suggestions of favoured methods and protocols from both those for whom microtechnique is a profession, as well as those who make microscopical preparations in their spare time.

Jeremy B. Sanderson
Oxford 1994

Acknowledgements

I have been fortunate to have the services of my colleagues in the Royal Microscopical Society, Dr Brian Bracegirdle and Dr Savile Bradbury. Dr Bracegirdle very kindly reviewed, commented on, and improved the clarity of the initial manuscript; many of his suggestions have been incorporated. Dr Bradbury, as General Editor of this series, has not only read and advised on the text, but also helped with the line diagrams, and instructed and encouraged me in developing my skills in microscopy.

I also wish to thank Dr Henry Teed for the production of many of the half-tone illustrations in this book, and whose support has been generously given. Several companies and societies have given permission for the use of their pictures; they are acknowledged in place, and I am grateful to the individuals concerned. My thanks are due to colleagues in the Department of Human Anatomy, the Nuffield Department of Surgery, as well as in my present Department, the Sir William Dunn School of Pathology, for their aid in the production of this book. I am indebted to Mr Douglas T. Richardson who has also read the manuscript. It is my pleasure to record my thanks to BIOS Scientific Publishers for their help.

This book has been greatly facilitated by the unstinted support of my wife, Yvonne. She not only read and commented upon the manuscript, but in addition managed a busy young family (largely unaided) until it was completed.

Safety

Attention to safety aspects is an integral part of all laboratory procedures and both the Health and Safety at Work Act and the COSHH regulations impose legal requirements on those persons planning or carrying out such procedures.

In this and other Handbooks every effort has been made to ensure that the recipes, formulae, and practical procedures are accurate and safe. However, it remains the responsibility of the reader to ensure that the procedures which are followed are carried out in a safe manner and that all necessary COSHH requirements have been looked up and implemented. Any specific safety instructions relating to items of laboratory equipment must also be followed.

Contents

Abbreviations   xv

1. Introduction   1

Collecting material for specimen preparation   3
Choice of preparative technique   5
Looking at preparations   8
References   10

2. Fixation   11

Function and use of fixatives   11
Methods of fixation   14
   Immersion fixation   14
   Perfusion fixation   15
   Vapour fixation   16
   Phase-partition fixation   16
   Mechanical methods   17
When not to use fixation   17
The penetration of fixatives   17
Osmolarity and pH   18
Fixing agents   19
   Formaldehyde   19
   Glutaraldehyde and acrolein   20
   Alcohols and acetone   21
   Mercuric chloride   21
   Potassium dichromate   21
   Picric acid and acetic acid   22
   Osmium tetroxide   22
Fixative mixtures   22
Secondary fixation   29
Preservatives   29
Washing tissues   29
Microwaves in histology   30
Microwaving formalin-fixed tissues   32
   Leiden fixative   34

ix

Microwaving paraffin sections   34
Microwaving cryostat sections   34
Staining reactions   35
Safety   35
References   35

3. Tissue Processing   39

Dehydration   41
Transition media   42
Processing schedules   43
Automatic processing   44
Embedding media   46
   Wax embedding   46
Preparation for cutting   50
Ribboning   51
   Ribboning difficulties   52
   Laying out ribbons   52
Mounting sections onto slides   52
   The water-bath method   53
   The hot-plate method   54
Marking slides   55
   Locating unstained sections   55
Storing wax blocks   56
Rehydrating sections   56
Gelatin-based embedding media   57
Other embedding media   58
Polyethylene glycol (PEG) waxes   58
Polyester waxes   59
   Ester wax   59
   Polyester wax   59
Cellulose embedding   60
   Double embedding   61
Orientation of small objects whilst embedding   62
Resin embedding media   63
   Epoxy resins   65
   Acrylic resins   67
   Lowicryl and London resins   70
Resin removal   72
Methods for hard tissues   72
   Decalcification   73
   Determination of end-point   74
   Sectioning   75
   Wax impregnation   76
   Resin impregnation   76
Lignified tissues   76
Insect tissues   78

Hair fibres   79
Diatom frustules   79
Recording tissue processing   80
References   80

4. Microtomy   85

Types of microtome   85
  Hand microtome   85
  Cambridge rocking microtome   85
  Rotary microtomes   86
  Base-sledge and sliding microtomes   87
  Freezing microtome   88
  Automated microtomes   89
Clamps and chucks   89
Types of knives   90
  Important knife angles and bevels   92
  Facets   93
  Care of knives   94
  Disposable blades   94
  Glass and diamond knives   95
Cryotomy   96
  Cold knife methods   96
  Cryostats   97
Freezing   97
  Embedding   99
  Hazards of cryogenic fluids   99
  Orientation of tissue   100
Cryostat sectioning   101
  Sectioning temperatures   102
  Anti-roll plate   102
  Electrostatic charges   102
  Handling sections   104
  Storage of tissue   104
Knife sharpening   105
  Lubricants   106
  Types of abrasive   107
  Handles and backs   107
  Manual sharpening   108
  Lapping   109
  Stropping   109
Sectioning   111
  Wax structure   112
  Compression   113
  Clearance angle   116
  Sectioning technique   116
Section thickness   119

Cryostat sectioning   120
Effect of fixation and processing on tissue size   120
Sectioning difficulties   123
  Softening fluids   124
  Static   124
  Summary   125
Vibratomes (tissue choppers)   125
  Macrotomes   131
Freehand sectioning   132
References   133

5. Other Preparative Methods   137

Cytological methods   137
Cytological fixatives   138
Cytocentrifuging and sedimentation   139
  Adherence and loss of cells   141
Smears   142
Imprints and replicas   142
  Cell blocks   144
Squashes   145
  Maceration   145
Temporary mounts   146
  Irrigation   146
Preparations of whole mounts in cells or 'boxes'   147
  Dry mounts   148
  Fluid mounts   151
Gum media   154
  Glycerol jelly mounts   154
  Glycerol fluid mounts   157
  References   157

6. Staining and Dyeing   159

Nomenclature   159
Staining action   160
  Mordants   161
  Metachromasia   162
Nuclear stains   163
  Haematoxylin   163
  Differentiation   165
  'Blueing'   165
  Other nuclear stains   165
  Carmine   166
  Safranin   166
  Synthetic nuclear dyes   166
Counterstains   166

Eosin	167
Other counterstains	167
General staining procedures	167
Selected staining protocols	170
Stains for glycerol jelly mounts	171
Stains for resin-embedded material	172
Block staining	173
Multiple staining of sections	173
Cytological stains	174
Neutral stains	174
Papanicolaou stain	177
Polychrome stains	179
Vital stains	183
Staining for bacteria	184
Removal of intrinsic pigments	186
Formalin and malarial pigments	186
Mercury pigment	187
Picric acid	187
Osmium tetroxide	187
Dye purity	187
References	188

7. Finishing the Preparation   191

Mountants	191
Water-based media	191
Dehydration and clearing	192
Resinous media	193
Mounting technique	194
Coverslip thickness	195
Adhesives	198
Lifting of sections	199
Cleaning slides	200
Fading of specimens	201
Sections stained with fluorochromes	202
Finishing the preparation	202
Using a ringing table	203
Labelling	205
Transport	205
Artifacts	207
Restoring preparations	209
Repairing broken slides	209
Restaining faded sections	210
Restoring tissues dried during processing	210
References	211

Appendices

Appendix A: Safety   213
Appendix B: Refractive indices   217

Index   219

Abbreviations

BDMA	benzyl dimethylamine
BPO	benzoyl peroxide
COSHH	Control of Substances Hazardous to Health
cP	centipoise
CRAF	chromo-acetic-formalin
DABCO	1, 4-diazo-bicyclo-(2,2,2)-octane
DBP	dibutyl phthalate
DDSA	dodecenyl succinic anhydride
DGD	diglycol distearate
DMA	$N'N$-dimethylaniline
DMP	2,2 dimethoxy-propane
DMP-30	2,4,6-tris(dimethylaminomethyl)phenol
DMSO	dimethyl sulphoxide
EDTA	ethylenediaminetetra-acetic acid disodium salt
FAA	formol-acetic-alcohol
FNAB	fine needle aspiration biopsy
FWA	Flemming without acetic
GMA	glycol methacrylate
HEMA	2-hydroxyethylmethacrylate
H & E	haematoxylin and eosin
IMS	industrial methylated spirits
LVN	low viscosity nitrocellulose
MMA	methyl methacrylate
NBS	Northern Biological Supplies
PEG	polyethylene glycol
PLP	periodate-lysine-paraformaldehyde
PTFE	polytetrafluoroeluene
PVP	polyvinylpyrrolidone
R-G	Romanowsky-Giemsa
RI	refractive index
TESPA	3-amino-propyl tri-ethoxy silane

1 Introduction

There are three basic methods for preparing biological material: smears, whole mounts and sections. These three can be further categorized into six distinct types (*Figure 1.1*). Fluid tissues, or suspensions of cells or tissues, may be studied directly as smears, cytospins or squashes between the slide and coverglass. Whole mounts tend to be used for small organisms, in a small cell built onto the slide topped with a coverglass. Examples of these preparations may be aquatic organisms in fluid mounts, insects in glycerol mounts or diatoms as dry mounts. Sections are used to study the internal cells and tissues of larger organisms. A rapid alternative to sectioning for studying the surface cells of organs is to take an impression.

The Royal Microscopical Society standardized the size of the glass slide at $3'' \times 1''$ (76×26 mm), or $3'' \times 1.5''$ (76×38 mm) in the middle of the nineteenth century, and most preparations are usually confined to these dimensions. Hydrated biological material must be treated with fixatives to prevent decay and preserve shape during subsequent treatment of naturally soft tissue, since most specimens are examined in the non-living state. This is an almost universal requirement; an obvious exception is the siliceous diatom frustule which remains after digestion of the living protoplasm.

Early workers studied both living and dead tissue, but nowadays supravital staining of living tissue is limited to the selective staining of certain cell components, or to the more recent use of injected intravital tracer dyes. The greater the number of steps in a preparative technique, the greater the number of artifacts which can be introduced. The production of artifacts is inevitable: death itself is an artifact of the living state. The normal status of the tissue or organism which we are studying can be assessed by comparing examples prepared in different ways, but it is important to recognize and understand why artifacts occur.

Most preparations are mounted between glass because a transparent support is required for transmitted light microscopy and a flat cover of glass forms part of the optical system for corrected objectives. Plastic coverglasses are used in tissue culture for temporary purposes, but these scratch easily, so for permanent preparations glass is essential. Glass, however, has two major disadvantages: it is fragile and prone to breakage, and materials adhere to it with difficulty. This has led to the development

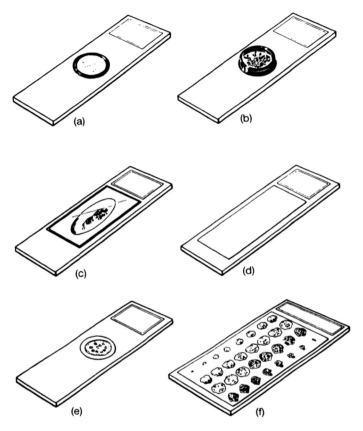

Figure 1.1:   Types of microscopical preparation. Preparations (a), (b) and (c) are whole mounts, either mounted strewn in mountant (a); as a dry or fluid mount (b); a whole mount or macerated preparation (c). Slide (d) shows a smear or imprint. Preparations of a single section (e) and serial sections (f) are illustrated. Reproduced from Gray (1954).

of special glues, as well as multi-step protocols for making whole mounts and fluid mounts. It is possible to avoid using glass, and to construct instead metal or wooden supports for opaque preparations examined using reflected light (Gray, 1954).

Biological specimen preparation is a conservative art, and most of the methods used today were in general use by the end of the nineteenth century. Modern methods of localizing cells and cellular components of interest, such as immuno-staining, have largely been adapted to suit time-honoured methods of preparing tissues. Prior to the nineteenth century most preparations were confined to dried specimens or temporary wet mounts. Thin pieces of tissue were held between slips of mica and inserted, in series, into a wooden slider. The historical development of preparative techniques has been fully described by Bracegirdle (1986, 1989).

The final image quality of the preparation for the microscope, and the conclusions drawn from it, depends upon many factors. Values determined for erythrocyte diameter will serve as an example. The human erythrocyte is normally about 7.8 µm in diameter *in vivo*, and 7.2–7.5 µm in blood smears. This value can range from 6 to 10 µm in sections, depending upon how the tissue has been preserved. Fixing and drying may shrink the cell due to water loss; in general, smear preparations result in a larger, flatter, cell than sections. Allowance may also have to be made for the age, and physiological or environmental status of the tissue at the moment a biopsy, or sample, is taken. Erythrocyte diameter is reduced in the case of iron-deficient anaemias; under conditions of folic acid deficiency it is increased. High altitude can alter erythrocyte diameter, as can the genotype of the organism. Further, these values given refer to human blood. There are often differences between similar tissues taken from different species. Measuring technique, including the accuracy of the calibration standard used for measurement, can vary and also influence the result. Micrometric methods are explained in Handbook 23 in this series (Bradbury, 1991). The erythrocyte is plastic, and can deform temporarily to traverse the micro-capillary network. In sections we view the shape assumed and caught at the time of sampling.

1.1 Collecting material for specimen preparation

Most workers wishing to prepare material for microscopy will study a limited range of organisms, and already be familiar with raising, culturing or collecting the species in question because of their research interests or adopted field of study. For those new to microscopy who have not yet defined a field of interest, it is suggested that they read a practical introductory text such as that of Gravé (1991).

The diversity and abundance of animal, plant and microbial life available for collection means that gathering material can be a relatively simple task. Nevertheless, a methodical approach ensures that specimens are less likely to suffer damage and full details of their natural habitat are known, which will place any serious study into scientific context. Concomitant with the proper collection of material is an understanding of taxonomy. Readers wishing to know more about this subject are advised to consult Jeffrey (1989) and Margulis and Schwartz (1988). For our purposes, we can regard specimens as aquatic, static terrestrial (in general, plants) and mobile terrestrial forms. These notes are confined to remarks on collecting microbial, herbaceous or invertebrate life from the wild. Subculturing and propagating research material, or raising chordate populations, requires special facilities and is beyond the scope of this text.

A variety of microbes can be cultured using a simple hay infusion. A handful of chopped grass can be added to tap water that has previously been allowed to stand for a day or so to remove the chlorine, and after a few days bacteria will accumulate. The culture can be further enriched by the addition of horse manure. Likewise, animal pellets and soil samples can be collected and dissected into water or buffer to provide material for investigation.

Botanical specimens can be collected into polythene bags, or kept pressed between two lightweight boards lined with paper. In humid climates collection in alcohol vapour is preferred to prevent decay. Alternatively, specimens can be dissected and immersion-fixed in the field. Likewise, fungi can usually be dissected into small cubes for fixation in the field. Spore samples can be taken as imprints from the fruiting body (Section 5.5) by placing the hymenial surface directly onto the slide and fixed by air drying. Further details for collecting botanical specimens can be found in Forman and Bridson (1992).

Many insects live and feed on plants; they can be beaten or shaken into an umbrella or net, or else picked or sucked off with an aspirator. Insects are best killed using a bottle containing a swab soaked in ethyl acetate, or cyanide, or by immersion into 70% alcohol (which also fixes the specimen). Some insects are phototropic and can be caught using a light trap, while others respond to chemical repellents or attractants. Those insects which inhabit woodland floor detritus can be sifted using Tüllgren or Berlèse funnels. Further details are given in Borror *et al.* (1989), in addition to the guides published by the Natural History Museum for collectors of insects and other invertebrates.

Aquatic invertebrate species can be collected directly in glass vials or screw-top jars, or dredgings from plankton nets taken to provide species trapped in the algal weed. Benthic animals can be dislodged by stirring the water and overturning stones upstream of the net. Empty the contents of the net into a white dish, or translucent container with a white sheet or paper background. The animals will at once crawl out from the detritus, and can be identified and selected. Sorting is much easier if living forms are sorted; when dead they resemble the dredgings and, lacking movement, are much harder to discriminate. Many invertebrates will survive transport amongst damp weed kept in an air-tight tin better than they will in overcrowded bottles of water. If bottles are used, they should be cleaned with only a small amount of detergent and rinsed several times with tap water. Just prior to use, rinse out the bottle with pond water before sampling. When filling bottles, they should be left two thirds empty to provide a sufficiently high surface area to volume ratio between the water and air.

Whatever the species collected, a hard-backed notebook should be used to record in pencil (later written up in ink) details of the collection, identified and suspected species, locality, weather, temperature and date. Details of suitable field record sheets, and further details of collection can be found in Needham (1962), Garnett (1965) and Knudsen (1972).

For initial identification and selection of material a good 10× hand lens (preferably with an achromatic doublet) is indispensable. Where it is imperative to keep both hands free (e.g. dissection) use an eye loupe, or magnifier fitted to a head band. Should higher magnifications be required there are two portable field microscopes on the market. The classical McArthur microscope is manufactured by W. Kirk & Sons, and can be adapted for use with phase, fluorescence and other contrast techniques. The Lensman microscope (Alltek Precision Plastics) is constructed of plastic and, while not of the same quality as the McArthur design, is much cheaper. Besides these instruments, it is possible to use microscopical video equipment, and minature microscopes with long working distances. For further details, see Watt (1993).

1.2 Choice of preparative technique

There may be sufficient tissue to compare the results of several different preparative techniques, but often, particularly in the case of clinical biopsies, tissue is scarce. The decision may then have to be taken whether to snap-freeze labile tissue for frozen section cryotomy, or to select the appropriate fixative for paraffin sectioning and the demonstration of a particular cell constituent.

The prime considerations in the choice of technique are what is being studied and the questions that require answering. It is also important to consider whether material must be stored or sent to colleagues. The equipment available may also determine whether a particular (e.g. fluorescence, confocal) technique can be used.

It is often useful, and time-saving, to decide whether to use the light microscope or electron microscope at the outset of study. The light microscope is extremely versatile, and Hillman and Richards (1983) give a review of the basic light microscope techniques available, but for the study of ultrastructure or surface detail the transmission or scanning electron microscope may well prove superior. It is possible to prepare tissue so that it can be examined by both modes, but this is not usual, and involves compromise. The wisest course is to decide on the method of examination and preparation beforehand. *Table 1.1* compares the relative merits of each method of microscopical examination. For examination of the same tissue sample by light and electron microscopy the reader is referred to Hayat (1987).

Table 1.1:   Comparison between light and electron microscopy

Advantages	Disadvantages	Notes
Light Microscopy		
Living tissue may be examined	Contrast is often low, specimen may move!	Most tissue, however, is examined dead and fixed
Low magnification possible	Maximum magnification 1400 times	Limited magnification compared to EM
Wide field of view available	Limited field of view at high magnifications	
Long working distance possible	Resolution limited by long working distance and large depth of focus (when present)	Conventional binocular system usually has small depth of field and depth of focus
Operates close to physical limit of resolution	Resolution limited by wavelength of light to about 0.25 μm	Improvements possible by video and confocal scanning methods
Serial sectioning, confocal and deconvolution techniques permit 3-D reconstruction	Specimen thickness and objective numerical aperture limit vertical resolution	Optical sectioning possible
Versatile, cheap, easy to set up, service and use.	Less automated than EM. Proper alignment imperative for useable images	Many interchangeable accessories available
Wide range of analytical and measuring techniques are available	The unaided eye is bad at estimation	Computer-aided image analysis techniques obviate labour-intensive error-prone methods
Many methods of introducing contrast are possible	Contrast is usually low in routine brightfield with unstained material	
Non-invasive coloured optical staining possible	Modern microscope stands may not have substage filter holders	e.g. Rheinberg illumination, dispersion staining
Coloured staining with dyes easy	Selectivity often difficult	Histochemical and immunohistochemical staining improve selectivity
Preparations relatively quick and simple to make	Preparations generally crude at ultrastructural level	

Table 1.1: *continued*

Advantages	Disadvantages	Notes
Electron Microscopy		
Greater resolving power (1 nm)	Lens quality and specimen preparation limit resolving power	Major aberrations cannot be cancelled out
High magnifcation (up to 500,000 times) compared to LM	Limited field of view	Image may rotate as the magnification is changed
SEM has large depth of field and depth of focus over all magnifications. Depth of field 500–1000 greater than LM	TEM has very small depth of field and depth of focus	STEM instruments can combine both advantages
SEM has long working distance	TEM has short working distance	
Serial sectioning permits 3-D reconstruction	Confocal techniques not possible	Serial sectioning very difficult and tedious
More automated than LM. Good images possible from basic operation	Expensive to run and maintain, requires frequent alignment and specialist servicing	
Wide range of analytical and measuring techniques outside visible range of electromagnetic spectrum possible	Unable to exploit coloured wavelengths of visible range of the electromagnetic spectrum	X-rays radiated by specimen may be collected and analysed (e.g. elemental analysis, diffraction techniques)
Good staining from heavy metal stains	Methods of introducing contrast are generally limited	
TEM samples must usually be very thin sections or suspensions	Labour-intensive and time-consuming to prepare. Specimens very fragile, difficult to store	
EM specimen preparations usually have fewer artifacts	Ultrastructural studies demand higher quality of preparation	
SEM samples generally easy and quick to prepare	SEM specimens must be conducting or coated	
	Instrument normally operates under high vacuum. Living tissue will not survive	Wet SEM methods possible

LM, light microscope; EM, electron microscope; SEM, scanning electron microscope; TEM, transmission electron microscope.

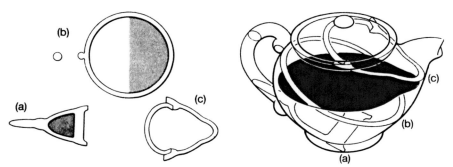

Figure 1.2:   Interpreting preparations. View of an entire teapot and three sections (a, b, c) in different planes. Cavities (if they are not filled) and vessels may present differing appearances according to how the section is cut. Reproduced from Rogers (1983) *Cells and Tissues* with permission from Academic Press.

1.3 Looking at preparations

The best prepared specimen will fail to give the information required if the instrument is not properly set up to begin with. Reference should be made to the first Handbook in this series, *An Introduction to the Optical Microscope* (Bradbury, 1989), to emphasize this crucial point.

A methodical approach to studying any preparation will reveal the maximum information in a quick, efficient and orderly way. This is particularly true of sections (Chapter 4) where it may be confusing to visualize structures in only two dimensions, as shown in *Figures 1.2* and *1.3*. The overall picture may be further distorted by artifacts, and cell components may be lost in processing (for example, lipid loss during infiltration with paraffin prior to sectioning).

Do not immediately use the high magnification objectives to look at your preparation. The greater the magnification used, the less the depth of focus and the smaller the field of view. Study the preparation using the unaided eye, a hand lens and the lowest power objectives first, to provide information to which the limited views at higher magnification can be related. The advice given by Henry Baker in *The Microscope Made Easy* (1742) is still pertinent:

> When you employ the microscope, shake off all prejudice, nor harbour any favourite opinions; for, if you do, 'tis not unlikely fancy will betray you into error, and make you see what you would wish to see.

Chapter 6 deals with preparing cytological material for examination where the reduction from three dimensions to the two seen in the final preparation is by means different from sectioning. Populations of cells are spread on the slide by smears, imprints or cytocentrifuging. These cells are not held together in a connective tissue matrix in the same way as cells in tissue biopsies, and so may have altered morphology, or lost cytoplasm, as

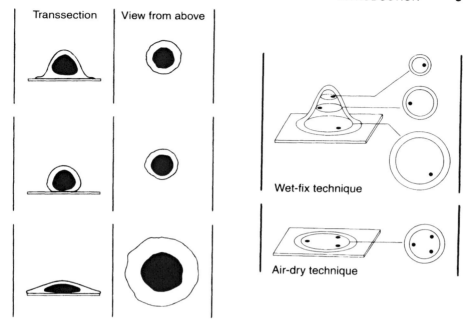

Figure 1.3: Interpreting preparations. Comparison of two-dimensional cell morphology seen following various different cytological preparation techniques (left). The influence of cytopreparatory technique on the localization of cellular organelles (right). The organelles seen in the single plane of focus of the flat air-dried cell, will require careful focusing to be seen by a high numerical aperture objective in the three planes in which they are located in the taller wet-fixed cell. Reproduced from Boon and Drijver (1985) *Routine Cytological Staining Techniques: Theoretical Background and Practice* with permission from Macmillan Press Ltd.

a result of exfoliation or damage during collection. Likewise, preferential groups of cells may be collected for sampling, or subsequently lost during preparation. Isolated cells are more prone to damage and morphological change than cells held *in situ* within a block of tissue.

The range of techniques available to biologists is very large, and cannot be covered in an introductory book of this size. For general animal histology the reader is referred to Bancroft and Stevens (1990), and for plant histology to Purvis, Collier and Walls (1966) and Berlyn and Miksche (1976). Gray's *Microtomist's Formulary and Guide* (1954) and *Peacock's Elementary Microtechnique* (Bradbury, 1973) are classics in micro-technique that stand apart. Although staining protocols are given later in this book, they serve merely to demonstrate selected principles, and the reader is referred to *H.J. Conn's Biological Stains* (Lillie, 1977), Clark (1981) and Cook (1974) for a more complete treatment.

There is a range of specialist journals: pre-eminent amongst these was *Stain Technology*, now renamed *Biotechnic and Histochemistry*. Other journals worth consulting are *Histochemistry and Cytochemistry, Histochemistry, Journal of Immunological Methods, Micron, Journal of Micro-*

scopy, and *The Quekett Journal of Microscopy* (formerly *Microscopy*). *Microscope* and the *Transactions of the American Microscopical Society*, in the USA, have useful articles. Two other relevant journals, which have been renamed, are *Microscopica Acta* (now merged with *Micron*) and the *British Journal of Biomedical Science* (formerly *Medical Laboratory Sciences*).

References

Bancroft JD, Stevens A. (eds) (1990) *Theory and Practice of Histological Techniques*, 3rd edn. Churchill Livingstone, Edinburgh.

Berlyn GP, Miksche JP. (1976) *Botanical Microtechnique and Cytochemistry*. Iowa State University Press, Ames, IA.

Borror DJ, Triplehorn CA, Johnson NF. (1989) *An Introduction to the Study of Insects*, 6th edn. Saunders, Philadelphia, PA.

Bracegirdle B. (1986) *A History of Microtechnique*, revised edn. Science Heritage, Lincolnwood, IL.

Bracegirdle B. (1989) The development of biological preparative techniques for light microscopy. *J. Microsc.* **155**, 307–318.

Bradbury S. (1973) *Peacock's Elementary Microtechnique*, 4th revised edn. Edward Arnold, London.

Bradbury S. (1989) *An Introduction to the Optical Microscope*, revised edn. Royal Microscopical Society Handbook No. 1, Oxford University Press, Oxford.

Bradbury S. (1991) *Basic Measurement Techniques for Light Microscopy*. Royal Microscopical Society Handbook No. 23, Oxford University Press, Oxford.

Bridson D, Forman I. (eds) (1992) *The Herbarium Handbook*, revised edn. Kew, London.

Clark G. (1981) *Staining Procedures*. Biological Staining Commission, William & Wilkins, Baltimore, MD.

Cook HC. (1974) *Manual of Histological Demonstration Techniques*. Butterworths, London.

Garnett WJ. (1965) *Freshwater Microscopy*, 2nd edn. Constable, London.

Gravé V. (1991) *Using the Microscope*. Dover, New York.

Gray P. (1954) *The Microtomist's Formulary and Guide*. Blakiston, New York.

Hayat MA. (ed.) (1987) *Correlative Microscopy in Biology: Instrumentation and Methods*. Academic Press, London.

Hillman H, Richards PR. (1983) Types of light microscopy. *Microscopy* **34**, 630–636.

Jeffrey C. (1989) *Biological Nomenclature*, 3rd edn. Edward Arnold, London.

Lillie RD. (1977) *H.J. Conn's Biological Stains*, 9th edn. Williams & Wilkins, Baltimore, MD.

Knudsen JW. (1972) *Preserving Plants and Animals*, Harper & Row, New York, London.

Margulis L, Schwartz, KV. (1988) *Five Kingdoms*, WH Freeman, New York.

Needham PR. (1962) *A Guide to the Study of Freshwater Biology*. Constable, London.

Purvis MJ, Collier DC, Walls D. (1966) *Laboratory Techniques in Botany*. Butterworths, London.

Watt IM. (1993) Light microscopes for use in unorthodox situations. *Microsc. Anal.* **38**, 27–29.

2 Fixation

2.1 Function and use of fixatives

Most biological specimens are examined in a non-living state. Such material must be stabilized, or fixed, for the following reasons.

(i)   Cellular and structural components must be kept as close as possible to the living state, and the tissue protected against osmotic shock, distortion and undue shrinkage.

(ii) Solution and loss of proteins, carbohydrates and other cell constituents must be minimized during subsequent processing.

(iii) Autolysis, fungal and bacterial decay must be arrested to avoid unacceptable artifacts.

(iv) The tissue must then be chemically prepared for differential staining to improve contrast and component demonstration.

(v)   The tissue must be hardened to allow subsequent processing and sectioning with the minimum of damage. In this case a decision must be made to 'trade-off' chemical alteration against mechanical damage.

(vi) Fixation alters the refractive index of tissue components, improving contrast if they are to be examined without staining.

Artifacts are unavoidable, and ensue immediately after death or excision of tissue from the living body. It may be helpful to regard the action of a fixative as similar to that of a camera: a 'picture' of the cell is taken which is as lifelike as possible. Autolysis (enzymic self-destruction) is accelerated at 37°C, and inhibited by extremes of heat or cold. Autolysis will disrupt the digestive system, for example, more than connective tissue or an insect whole mount which is largely chitinous. Autolytic changes may be recognized from the fragmentation, condensation and disappearance of cell nuclei. The cytoplasm becomes granular, eventually becoming a homogeneous swollen mass, without architecture or staining properties. Similar changes occur from the action of bacteria, especially in the gut. It is necessary to ensure rapid and immediate fixation in these cases. *Figure 2.1* shows an overview of the various steps in preparing biological

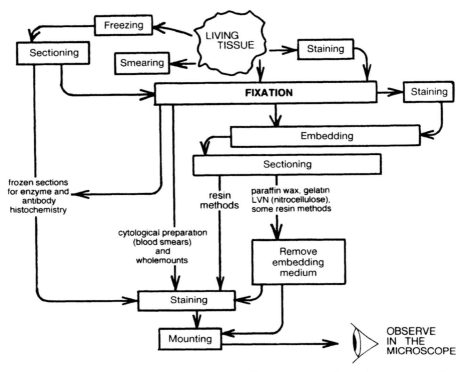

Figure 2.1: Preparing biological specimens. The sequence of specimen preparation, showing the central place of fixation. Reproduced from Horobin (1982) with permission from Gustav Fischer Verlag.

specimens for microscopical examination, and emphasizes the central place of fixation.

Fixation, although necessary, is all in all a rather drastic procedure, and perfect fixation is not possible, there being no universal fixative. Hence, a large number of mixtures have evolved for demonstrating particular organisms, tissues and cellular components. There have been few good studies on the suitability of different fixatives for various animal and plant tissues. The reader is referred to Stickland (1975) for muscle, which is a difficult tissue to fix; to Howard *et al.* (1989) for embryonic tissues, and Johnson *et al.* (1978) for the rat.

The function of fixatives is therefore to stabilize the tissue, most of which is protein. This is achieved by cross-linking end-groups of amino acids and coagulating the secondary and tertiary structures of proteins to form insoluble gels. The effects of fixatives on tissue size and tonicity is considered later, but is largely determined by how the fixative acts. Broadly speaking, histological fixatives may be divided into two groups, and the following list is largely taken from Culling *et al.* (1985).

1 Micro-anatomical fixatives

Allen's B-15
Bouin's
B-5 (formol-sublimate variant)
Formol-acetic-alcohol (FAA)
Formalin-alcohol
Formalin
Formol-saline and calcium
Formol-sublimate
Formol-sucrose
Heidenhain's SUSA
Gendre's
Glutaraldehyde, buffered
Rossman's
Zenker's
Zenker-formol (Helly's fluid)

2 Cytological fixatives

Nuclear
Carnoy's
Carnoy–Lebrun's
Clarke's
Flemming's
Navashin's
Newcomer's
Lewitsky–Baker's
Randolph's
  chromo-acetic-formalin (CRAF)
Sanfelice's

Cytoplasmic
Alcohol-based sprays
Champy's
Ether-alcohol
Formol-saline and calcium
von Orth's
Régaud's
Schaudinn's
Zenker-formol (Helly's fluid)

Micro-anatomical fixatives preserve the components of organs, tissues and cells in spatial relation to one another, and are the histological fixatives in routine use. They are largely coagulant in action, but micro-anatomical fixatives may have mixtures of non-coagulant agents as well. Cytological fixatives preserve cellular components, and are usually non-coagulant. The gross tissue block may be best fixed in the middle or outer zones, from which portions may be taken for examination. To give an example, the micro-anatomical fixative acidified potassium dichromate (Zenker's fluid) acts similarly to chromic acid as a coagulant of cytoplasm and chromatin, but cell organelles such as mitochondria are destroyed. In the less acid cytoplasmic cytological fixative Helly's fluid (Zenker-formol) nucleoproteins are not fixed, but mitochondria are preserved. Most fixatives used for examination of cytological preparations are based on ethanol, and are considered separately in Chapter 5.

Fixatives used for light microscopy are primarily coagulant types, the proteins forming the ultrastructure of the cell are coagulated rather like the white of an egg on cooking. This is obviously unsuitable for electron microscopical examination of cell ultrastructure, and in these cases non-coagulant fixatives are used. Paraffin wax easily penetrates the spongy structure produced by coagulant fixatives to permit sectioning.

Non-coagulant fixatives convert the cytoplasm into an insoluble gel so that while cell organelles are preserved, penetration is poor and artifacts are more likely to occur. Sections from tissues fixed in coagulant fixatives are more likely to distort than those from non-coagulants. Plastic and acrylic resin embedding compounds cause less distortion than wax or nitrocellulose, and are now widely used in light microscopy.

The combined effect of coagulation and hardening helps to prevent lysis by hyper- or hypotonic solutions. Most lipids are preserved merely by avoiding solvents, rather than being affected directly by fixatives. Dissolution is prevented by the coagulation of associated proteins. Fixatives also contain a chromatin nucleoprotein coagulant to facilitate nucleic counterstaining, and fixation generally facilitates the entry of dyes into the section. Some fixatives act as mordants between stain and tissue; an example of this is the use of potassium dichromate before staining myelin with haematoxylin.

Where large amounts of a particular tissue are available, different portions may be treated for various protocols requiring different fixation, for example immunohistology, enzyme histochemistry and electron microscopy. Where a small amount of material from a single source only is available, a decision must be made as to which fixative is most suitable, as explained in Section 1.2.

The distinction between preservatives, fixatives and mountants is a fine one. A preservative must act to inhibit tissue destruction and permit storage; a fixative must do this, but also preserve morphology and histochemical activity in the face of subsequent processing for specimen preparation. Preservatives may be used for dissection, whole mounts or museum specimens, or for the storage of material for subsequent preparation and microscopical examination, either before or after fixation. A preservative differs from a mountant in that the latter will, of its own accord, hold a coverglass in place without sealing. Details of preservatives are given in Section 2.9, and mountants in Chapter 7.

2.2 Methods of fixation

2.2.1 Immersion fixation

Immersion is the simplest and most routinely used method of fixation. Tissues should be sliced, or diced into small blocks, and immersed in an excess of fixative (20 times the volume of the tissue) to ensure adequate and sufficiently rapid penetration. Samples should, preferably, be suspended by thread or laid on a bed of lint-free gauze to present the maximum surface area for diffusion of the fixative into the tissues. When using fixative mixtures, the constituents do not penetrate at the same rate as the individual primary fixatives; consequently, zones appear in the material, which can only equilibrate in a large volume of fixative. The optimum block size will vary according to the penetration rate of the fixative used. In general, tissue should be dissected into blocks between 2 and 4 mm across the narrowest face for light microscopy, and no more than 1 mm^3 for joint electron microscopy studies.

Histological dissection techniques differ from those used in anatomy. The aim of the histologist is to excise the tissue with the minimum of disruption in order to preserve integrity at the microscopical level, whereas the anatomist essentially peels and scrapes away the layers of connective tissue from the gross organs of interest. It is important, therefore, to work quickly with very sharp instruments and forceps without serrated edges, and to leave sufficient 'waste' matter around the tissue of interest so that it neither dries out nor is unduly damaged. Because fixatives act relatively slowly, large organs are best sliced or opened up and allowed a further period of fixation before taking tissue blocks. Furthermore, since unfixed tissue is difficult to restrain and dissect, an initial period of fixation will aid in taking tissue samples for further processing. Drury and Wallington (1980) and Hopwood (1990) give details of the best procedures to follow for specific tissues and organs

2.2.2 Perfusion fixation

Specimens may also be fixed by perfusion through the vasculature (usually of a whole animal, but also of an individual organ). Tissue is perfused for speed and fixation is completed by immersion. Perfusion allows very even fixation with slow penetrating fixative mixtures. Artifacts and tissue damage from autolysis, decay and handling during dissection are minimized. This is therefore the method of choice for electron microscopical studies. Perfusion is carried out under anaesthesia using the heart and gravity or positive pressure via a syringe to pump the fixative into the tissue. The pressure determines the speed of fixation, and should be sufficient to displace the blood, without being in vast excess of the physiological arterial pressure of the live animal. The usual range is from 100 to 120 mmHg; a bottle 120–250 cm above the perfusion table is sufficient for gravity perfusion. The height of the bottle depends upon the size of the animal: 120–160 cm for small, and 200–250 cm for large mammals. It is essential to pre-wash the vasculature free of blood otherwise the fixative causes clumping of erythrocytes and thrombosis. Allow 400 ml pre-wash solution per kilogram body weight, or perfuse until organ is grey-white. The pre-wash fluids may simply be 0.9% saline, Ringer's solution or fixative buffer, often with vasodilators (0.5% w/v procaine or 1 ml of 1% sodium nitrite), anti-coagulants (0.25% w/v heparin) or osmotically active colloids (dextran) added. The effect of dextran or polyvinylpyrrolidone (PVP) is to prevent the enlargement of extra-vascular spaces. Further details of suitable additives and the osmolarity of various tissues are given in the references at the end of this section.

Animals are either perfused newly dead, or under sufficiently deep anathaesia to avoid physiological stress and pain. Cut the costal cartilages, and sternum to expose the pericardium, which should be reflected back to expose the large arteries. Perfuse with a cannula from the left ventricle to right atrium, the aortic bifurcation, or arterial vasculature above the organ of interest. Drain the perfusate (about $2 \, l \, kg^{-1}$) through an incision in the right ventricle. Perfuse the animal with pre-wash fluid until it runs clear, and follow with the appropriate fixative until the animal is rigid. Following a good quality perfusion without thrombi, blood-rich organs will turn grey-white, and a slight muscle tremor will be seen. Dissect out the required tissues into ice-cold fixative and continue fixation by immersion at 4°C. Comprehensive accounts for perfusing frogs, rodents and large mammals are given in Ross (1972), Robinson *et al.* (1987), Hayat (1989) and Côté *et al.* (1993). A method involving precise perfusion controlled by a pressure-sensitive feedback loop has been published by Rostgaard *et al.* (1993).

2.2.3 Vapour fixation

This method is not much used, but is effective for thin or delicate tissues, or where expensive, volatile fixatives must be used such as osmium tetroxide and formaldehyde. Vapour fixation is usually employed to fix freshly cut cryostat sections, or freeze-dried tissue. Formaldehyde fumes (from hot paraformaldehyde) will fix tissue sections in 2 h at 70°C in a wax oven, or in a few minutes in a microwave oven. Vapour fixation is suitable for fixing moieties such as glycogen which will otherwise flow within the boundary of the cell with aqueous fixatives.

2.2.4 Phase-partition fixation

Another little-used method, phase-partition fixation, has been reported as suitable for reducing shrinkage of tissue which is fixed by immersion in an organic solvent in equilbrium with the aqueous fixative of choice. It is suited to small and delicate tissues susceptible to osmosis. Changes in tissue morphology and volume due to protein loss and distortion (by movement of water) are less than by conventional aqueous fixation alone. The success of the method depends very much upon the correct choice of solvent and fixative. Heptane and Omnisolve (1,1,2-trichlorotrifluoro-ethane) are good vehicles for 50% aqueous glutaraldehyde, in particular, and formaldehyde. Phase-partition fixation usually requires a greater concentration of fixative than aqueous immersion alone. For a comparison of this technique with aqueous fixation and further details on the optimum treatment of individual tissues, see Nettleton and McAuliffe (1986).

Phase-partition has also been useful for fixing mucus *in situ* on the surfaces of tissues (Sims *et al.*, 1991). This mucus layer is often washed away during conventional fixation and subsequent processing. Infiltration or post-fixation should usually be carried out under vacuum to remove all traces of fluorocarbon from the fixed tissues, which will otherwise interfere with the subsequent curing of plastic resins.

2.2.5 Mechanical methods

These include freezing and heating. Freezing is only a temporary physical process and must be followed by chemical fixation or removal of the water. It is often used where immunological or histochemical demonstration of labile components is required. Freeze substitution is most often employed in scanning electron microscopy to remove water by sublimation without incurring chemical insult from fixation or mechanical damage. The technical aspects are discussed by Harvey (1982). Freeze-dried tissue can also be prepared for resin and paraffin histology; details can be found in Murray and Ewen (1991). Classically, smears and blood films have been fixed by heat, but the direct application of dry heat is rarely used, being uneven and fierce in its action thereby disrupting cellular architecture. Wet-fixation methods give less erratic results, but if heat is used in conjunction with wet-fixation, it should not generally be applied above 60°C.

2.3 When not to use fixation

The successful fixation of fats, antigens and enzymes, and other complex protein structures such as chromosomes and nucleic acids have presented problems for clinicians and research workers alike. Fresh tissue is often required for clinical diagnosis and immunocytochemistry. In this case the tissue is cut while frozen and then lightly fixed, rather than collected and stored for any length of time in fixative prior to subsequent treatment. Another very specific approach is to coat unfixed tissue with a semi-permeable membrane (Chayen and Bitensky, 1991) which allows reagent molecules access to the tissue without loss.

2.4 The penetration of fixatives

Most fixatives that penetrate tissues quickly tend to be swelling agents; the converse is also true. Ethanol is the slowest penetrator, yet the fastest acting fixative, causing much shrinkage of tissues. Conversely, acetic acid, the fastest penetrator, fixes slowly and swells tissues. As a general rule, 24 h is sufficient for most rapidly acting fixatives, where the block thickness is not more than 5 mm. Tissues fixed in slower penetrators should be not more than 2 mm thick. For the majority of fixatives the depth of penetration is linearly related to the square root of fixation time: $d = k\sqrt{t}$. This is not the case for osmium tetroxide whose reaction products impede the further entry of fixative. Penetration rates can also alter significantly depending upon which tissue is being fixed, and further details can be found in Hopwood (1990) and Horobin (1982).

2.5 Osmolarity and pH

These parameters are of greater importance in electron microscopy than light microscopy. The aqueous phase of fixatives penetrates more rapidly than the solutes, causing hypotonic swelling of tissue. Small unreactive ions and molecules, such as chlorides, sulphates, dextran, sucrose and PVP, may be added to fixative mixtures to reduce the effect of osmosis. Once fixed, tissues are not susceptible to osmotic action, and tissues may be washed in water. Isotonic solutions (250–350 mOsm) are recommended for tissues required for enzyme histochemistry, but otherwise seem to confer no particular advantage. Grossly hypertonic fixatives cause shrinkage, while isotonic and hypotonic fixatives cause swelling of cells and poor ultrastructural fixation. For joint light/electron microscope studies it is best to use a slightly hypertonic solution around 500 mOsm, at which most fixatives appear to work best.

It is not always the case that hypertonic fixatives shrink tissues: acetic acid causes swelling. Conversely, picric acid, a hypotonic fixative, causes tissue shrinkage. Also, the effects of 10% buffered formalin fixation can be reversed, and tissues can still suffer osmotic shock after 24 h. In general, coagulant fixatives shrink tissue, and cross-linking fixatives cause swelling, without regard for speed of penetration, action or osmotic pressure. Note that in many cases the action of dehydration, transition and embedding reagents markedly alters the final tissue volume (Section 4.10).

With the exception of neutral-buffered formalin, glutaraldehyde and osmium tetroxide, which are most effective at about neutrality, all other fixatives are acidic mixtures. Buffering to pH 7.2–7.6 is especially important for formalin, which coagulates protein more slowly than other fixatives. A study on the effect of buffers on tissue ultrastructure has been made by Wood and Luft (1965). A further study has been made by Pentilla *et al.* (1975) of the effect of fixatives on normal and injured cells, and these authors recommend that 10% formalin should be buffered to 310 mOsm. A graph of the influence of sodium chloride, sucrose and glucose vehicles on fixative osmolarity has been published by Maser *et al.* (1967).

2.6 Fixing agents

Fixing agents include:

aldehydes:	formaldehyde, paraformaldehyde, glutaraldehyde, acrolein;
ketones:	acetone;
alcohols:	methanol, ethanol;
mineral acids:	acetic, picric (hydrochloric and sulphuric are less used);
mercury salts:	mercuric chloride;
chromium salts:	potassium dichromate, chromic acid.

The action of these individual agents (simple, or primary, fixatives) and their derivative mixtures are often little understood. The chemistry is complex, but has been well covered by Pearse (1980), Horobin (1982), Hopwood (1985) and Kiernan (1990). Kiernan includes references to sources detailing ionic and organic fixative agents not mentioned above.

2.6.1 Formaldehyde

Formaldehyde is a gas which dissolves in water to a maximum of 40% by weight, and is commercially available as a 37% saturated solution by volume. The concentrated solution decomposes to formic acid and water on storage, and the diluted formalin solution is usually stored over calcium carbonate chips, or used as neutralized formalin with buffered salts. Avoid addition of concentrated formalin to carbonates: the rapid evolution of carbon dioxide can present an explosion hazard. Methanol is added (10–15% of volume) as a stabilizer to inhibit polymerization. Any turbidity is due to the formation of paraformaldehyde, which must be removed before use by filtration. Polymerization will also occur more rapidly in neutralized formalin, and therefore buffer salts should be added just before use to the diluted stock solution.

By convention the term formalin refers to a dilution from the stock solution. The term formaldehyde should only be used for the neat stock, and not the diluted working solution. For example, 10% formalin (the usual dilution of the working fixative) contains 4% formaldehyde, not 10% formaldehyde, which would otherwise be 25% formalin (and too strong for normal use, resulting in excessively hard tissues). American manufacturers and authors tend to refer to the saturated formaldehyde solution as 40% formalin. Although there is a slight difference between the 40% solution by weight and the 37% solution by volume, due to the fact that some manufacturers sell according to different specifications, the difference is usually so slight as not to matter, unless very large volumes are being made up, or the investigation demands very precise formulation.

Formalin vapour is an irritant, and prolonged exposure can cause dermatitis. The recommended threshold limit value (occupational exposure limit) is two parts per million. Further aspects of the effects of formaldehyde on safety are discussed by Hopwood (1985).

Because formalin penetrates rapidly, but fixes tissues slowly, the optimum fixation period in 10% formalin is 7–10 days, although 1–2 days is the length of time most commonly used, being sufficient for routine clinical use. In solution formalin is hydrated to form methylene glycol with an equilibrium in favour of methylene glycol. Hence, if tissues are insufficiently fixed and placed after only a few hours in the dehydrating alcohols, the centre of the tissue block will show an 'alcohol' pattern of fixation with clumped chromatin and shrunken cytoplasm, because of inadequate cross-linking of the cellular architecture and subsequent washing out of the remaining formalin.

Prolonged fixation in acid formalin causes haematin pigment (Section 6.10.1) to be deposited as a red-brown granular, birefringent material, which can be avoided by the use of buffered fixatives. Improved cellular detail, reduced shrinkage and distortion, and the absence of formalin pigment have been reported when 2% phenol is added to the fixative. Hopwood *et al.* (1989) suggest the sequential use of buffered phenol-formaldehyde at pH 7.0 and pH 5.5 at 40°C followed by conventional paraffin processing. Other workers (Dapson, 1993) recommend using 1% zinc sulphate in unbuffered 10% formalin for improved cytomorphology and retrospective immunohistochemical studies. A formalin-based fixative widely used for preserving labile antigens in immunological studies is periodate-lysine-paraformaldehyde (PLP) devised by McLean and Nakane (1974). Two good reviews of the use of formaldehyde in histology, and its effects on tissue shrinkage have been published by Crawford and Barer (1951) and Fox *et al.* (1985).

The advantages of using formalin as a fixative are as follows.

(i)   It is cheap and easily available.
(ii)   It is stable and works under a broad variety of conditions.
(iii)   It can be used either as a fixative or preservative over a 10-fold range of concentration from 2 to 20%.
(vi)   It can be used with most tissues.
(v)   It penetrates tissues rapidly, but can initially be washed out and its effects reversed.
(vi)   It does not overfix, and therefore tissue is not rendered too hard for sectioning, even after a few days.
(vii)   Although a coagulant, formalin fixatives do not cause excessive clumping, and can be used for diagnostic electron microscope studies.

2.6.2 Glutaraldehyde and acrolein

These chemicals act as cytological rather than micro-anatomical fixatives like formalin. The tissue is hardened to a greater extent with glutaraldehyde (a slow penetrator) and wax sectioning is more difficult, the wax penetrating the cross-linked tissue less well than formalin-fixed specimens. Acrolein (a rapid penetrator) is useful for large blocks of tissue, or those covered with impenetratable substances such as chitin or a waxy cuticle. It can only be used in conjunction with other fixatives, usually as a 4% solution in 2% glutaraldehyde buffered with 0.1 M cacodylate buffer to pH 7.3. These fixatives are rarely used in light microscopy, but recent evidence (Uehara *et al.*, 1993) suggests that the addition of glutaraldehyde to paraformaldehyde gives an improved quality of signal in *in situ* hybridization. For further details concerning *in situ* hybridization protocols, the reader is referred to Handbook 27 in this series (Leitch *et al.*, 1994), Stahl and Baskin (1993) and Wilcox (1993).

2.6.3 Alcohols and acetone

Alcohols displace water from proteins, disrupting hydrogen bonds and causing hardening and excessive shrinking. Therefore, they are best used to fix smears, films and cryostat sections. Nucleoprotein is left intact, and most of the lipids are dissolved out of the tissue. Alcohols are highly coagulative, and disrupt morphology. Tissue preservation with acetone, also a dehydrating fixative, is likewise poor. Ice-cold acetone and alcohol are best used to preserve enzyme or antigen activity in sectioned cryostat material, as cryostat sectioning post-fixed material (particularly acetone) is difficult. A technique employing acetone fixation followed by methyl benzoate and xylene (Sato *et al.*, 1986) is claimed to preserve labile antigens in paraffin wax which have previously only been demonstrated in frozen tissue.

2.6.4 Mercuric chloride

This is a white, crystalline, very poisonous salt, soluble in water to 7%, and alcohol to 33%. Mercuric chloride is corrosive of metals, and implements should be dipped in molten wax before use. It penetrates rapidly, shrinks, but does not distort, and permits good staining of both nucleus and cytoplasm. Overexposure of tissue to the fixative will cause excessive hardening. Mercury pigment, which occurs with fixatives such as Zenker's, SUSA and Helly's, can be removed with alcoholic iodine (Section 6.10.2). Where mercuric chloride has been used as a fixative in an automatic processor, and is subsequently intended to process specimens for autoradiography, all reagents should be changed; otherwise residual mercuric chloride, which has been carried over, will interfere with the autoradiographs.

2.6.5 Potassium dichromate

A saturated aqueous solution contains 15% of the salt. The pH is critical to the action of this precipitating fixative. Above pH 3.8 cytoplasm is homogeneously fixed, as are mitochondria, but no nucleoprotein is preserved. Below pH 3.4 mitochondria are destroyed, and nucleus and cytoplasm are preserved. Like chromic acid, potassium dichromate should be washed out of tissue before proceeding to dehydration, to prevent insoluble green precipitates forming. Soft, solid tissues may become brittle and section badly in paraffin wax after exposure to potassium dichromate.

2.6.6 Picric acid and acetic acid

Used alone picric acid will shrink tissues, and will cause tissue maceration after prolonged exposure, even within wax-embedded blocks. Acetic acid is used largely to coagulate chromatin, and to offset the shrinkage effects of alcohol and picric acid; it will dissolve cytoplasmic granules.

2.6.7 Osmium tetroxide

This costly, volatile and dangerous fixative is nowadays seldom used in light microscopy, but is used as a combined fixative and stain by electron microscopists. The vapours are highly irritant, particularly to the corneal epithelium. It is very easily reduced by heat, light and organic contaminants, but pure aldehydes and acetone are exceptions. Fixation of tissue with osmium tetroxide reverses the affinity of tissue for anionic dyes; the tissue then may be stained by cationic dyes, demonstrating basiphilic, rather than acidophilic, substances. Osmium tetroxide may be used to stain unsaturated lipids in frozen sections. It is an excellent cytological fixative, with absence of distortion; but tissue is rendered crumbly, which becomes worse on embedding in wax, leading to cracking and formation of shrinkage spaces. It is a poor penetrator: typically 1 mm^3 blocks require 3 h immersion. Osmium tetroxide is often incorrectly refered to as osmic acid. Further details of its use may be found in Hayat (1989) and Kiernan (1990).

2.7 Fixative mixtures

Table 2.1 lists the composition of commonly used fixatives for botanical and zoological purposes and a complete list may be found in Gray (1954). Spirits such as gin or vodka may be used as improvized fixatives. De-icers and commercial hair sprays have also been suggested; however, hair sprays (which also contain colouring agents) and some de-icer formulations contain methanol, which tends to make tissues, especially those of insects, very brittle. They should therefore be avoided if at all possible.

Table 2.1:   Protocols for fixative mixtures

Formalin fixatives

10% neutral-buffered formalin

40% formaldehyde	100 ml
Sodium hydrogen phosphate	4 g
Disodium phosphate (anhydrous)	6.5 g
Tap water	900 ml

Into 100 ml of hot water dissolve the reagents in the order stated (the disodium salt is least soluble). Cool by adding 700 ml cold tap water, add the formaldehyde and make up to 1 l. If 10% formalin is made up unbuffered, neutralize the diluted fluid with calcium carbonate ('marble chips') in the container.

10% formol-saline

40% formaldehyde	100 ml
Sodium chloride	8.5 g
Tap water	750 ml

Mix and decant into a dark bottle with a layer of calcium carbonate chips on the bottom. There is some distortion (but no over-hardening) of tissues in this fixative, but it is a good general fixative suited to marine animals, tissues which are to be decalcified and secondary fixation.

Neutral-buffered formol-saline

Sodium di-hydrogen phosphate (anhydrous)	1.00 g
Di-sodium hydrogen phosphate (anhydrous)	1.63 g
Sodium chloride	8.50 g
40% formaldehyde	75 ml

Make up to 1000 ml with distilled water. Adjust the pH to 7.0 with 1 M sodium hydroxide.

Formol-sucrose

40% formaldehyde	10 ml
Sucrose	7.5 g
0.1–0.2 M phosphate buffer pH 7.4	to 1000 ml

This is an excellent fixative for preserving cytoplasmic and enzyme structure, and is often used at 4°C followed by buffered 4% paraformaldehyde fixation.

Formol-calcium

Baker (1950) advocated the addition of 2% calcium acetate to neutralize and buffer 10% formalin, but Drury and Wallington (1980, p. 49) found that calcium artifacts simulate false positive areas of calcification in tissues, and so do not recommend this fixative.

Formalin-alcohol

Absolute ethyl alcohol	58 ml
40% formaldehyde	4 ml
Distilled water	38 ml

This is good for pollen, woody anatomical material, and can be used as a preservative or indefinite storage medium. Fix for 15–60 min minimum, followed by a 70% alcohol wash; this fixative shrinks and hardens most tissues.

Table 2.1:   *continued*

FAA

40% formaldehyde	10 ml
Acetic acid (glacial)	3 ml
50% ethyl alcohol or ethanol	87 ml

A good, stable, general fixative for stems, roots and leaves. Material can be stored indefinitely in the mixture. Propionic acid can also be used instead of acetic acid to fix bryophytes and pteridophytes. Fix for at least 12 h followed by a 50% alcohol wash. If dehydrating in tertiary butyl alcohol, do not wash, but go to 50% *t*-butanol. FAA is not suited to cytological study, but is best for impervious material. Where very hard woody material is being fixed, increase the formaldehyde, and decrease the acetic acid. Over-fixation can lead to sectioning problems, as vascular tissue becomes much harder than the protoplasm. Thin leaves require 12 h, thick leaves 24 h, and woody material 1 week. Do not use as a storage medium where 10% mercuric chloride has been added to the mixture. Formol-propionic acid substituted for the acetic acid hardens material less than FAA. Some authorities use 70% ethanol.

Mercuric chloride fixatives

Formol-sublimate (mercuric chloride-formalin, Lendrum's)

Mercuric chloride (sat. aqueous—8%)	900 ml
40% formaldehyde	100 ml

This is a good micro-anatomical fixative, although tissues are shrunk to some extent. It is a good secondary fixative to follow formol-saline; acidic and metachromatic stains stain intensely after fixation in this mixture. The usual fixation period is 12–24 h, but this can be prolonged; tissues should be washed in 70% alcohol after fixation. Tissues become white in this fixative; some workers therefore add 2–3 drops of 1% (aq) acid fuchsin to see the tissue in the block. B-5 calls for the addition of 1.25 g of anhydrous, or 2.07 g trihydrate sodium acetate. B-4 (which is B-5 without formaldehyde) is recommended by Lillie and Fullmer (1976) for Paneth granules or histochemical reactions which must avoid formaldehyde. The pH of B-4 and B-5 is about 5.8–6.0.

Zenker's

Mercuric chloride	5 g
Potassium dichromate	2.5 g
Sodium sulphate	1 g
Distilled water	100 ml
Glacial acetic acid (added just before use)	5 ml

Fix blocks for 3–18 h, then wash well in running water. Remove mercury pigment. A good micro-anatomical fixative; erythrocytes are not well preserved, but it is good for sharp histological detail. The stock without acetic acid will keep indefinitely.

Helly's (Zenker-formol, Maximow's)

Replace the acetic acid in Zenker's just before use with 5 ml formaldehyde. A good cytological fixative for mammals, and also for haemopoetic tissues. It can be used as a secondary fixative after 10% formol-saline to improve preservation and staining. It is slower than Zenker's. Fix for 6–24 h, wash in running water, remove mercury pigment. For non-mammalian tissues use Lewitsky–Baker's which is a modification of Flemming's fixative. It is good for both nuclear and cytoplasmic detail, and tissues decalcify well after fixation. Some workers report that ribbons handle less well due to static, and sections are prone to lift off the slide whilst processing.

Table 2.1: *continued*

Salt Zenker's

Mercuric chloride	27 g
Potassium dichromate	15 g
Sodium chloride (6%)	30 g
Single distilled water	100 ml
Acetic acid, 1 M (added just before use)	25 ml

This variant is non-haemolytic. Fixation for 5 h is recommended by Lillie *et al.* (1973).

Heidenhain's SUSA

Mercuric chloride	45 g
Sodium chloride	5 g
Trichloroacetic acid	20 g
Acetic acid (glacial)	40 ml
40% formaldehyde	200 ml
Distilled water	800 ml

A good fixative for biopsy material or invertebrates, but the red blood cells are not well preserved; many workers prefer the simpler formol-sublimate. Fix for 3–24 h; do not wash (which causes swelling of collagen), but transfer directly to 95% alcohol. It is a good cytoplasmic fixative, but over-fixation hardens tissues.

Chromic/dichromic fixatives
Sanfelice's

Solution A	40% formaldehyde	128 ml
	Acetic acid (glacial)	16 ml
Solution B	1% chromic acid	100 ml

Add 9 ml solution A to 16 ml solution B immediately before use. Fix thin blocks (less than 3 mm thick) for 12–24 h, followed by a wash in running water. Very good for chromosome studies.

Randolph's modified Navashin's Fluid (CRAF)

Solution A	Chromic acid	1 g
	Acetic acid (glacial)	7 ml
	Distilled water	92 ml
Solution B	10% formalin	30 ml
	Distilled water	70 ml

Mix equal quantities just before using, and fix the material for 12–24 h. Wash afterwards in several changes of 70% alcohol before dehydrating. It is used principally for smears and root-tip squashes.

Chrome-acetic (similar to Navashin's fluid)

10% (aq) chromic acid	2.5 ml	7.0 ml	10.0 ml
10% (aq) acetic acid	5.0 ml	10.0 ml	30.0 ml
Distilled water	92.5 ml	83.0 ml	60.0 ml

Use the weaker mixture (left) for more delicate materials, such as algae and fungi; the medium mixture (centre) for compact tissues; the strong mixture (right) for tough botanical tissues. Fix for 24 h, and wash thoroughly in running water.

Table 2.1:   *continued*

Flemming's fixative

1% (aq) chromic acid	15 ml
2% (aq) osmium tetroxide	4 ml
Acetic acid (glacial)	0.5–1 ml

This is best used as a secondary fixative for myelin. Fix small blocks of tissue for 12–48 h, and transfer to running water.

Flemming without acetic (FWA)

2% (aq) osmium tetroxide	4 ml
1% (aq) chromic acid	15 ml

This should be made up fresh, and small tissue blocks fixed for 24 h. After a thorough wash in tap water for up to 6 h, dehydration should proceed from 30% alcohol. The fixative can be made isotonic with sodium chloride at 3% for marine organisms and 0.8% for others.

Lewitsky–Baker's

Prepare FWA with 0.75% (aq) sodium chloride as the solvent. Drury and Wallington (1980) claim it is superior for cytoplasmic organelles. Fix for 12–24 h. It is best for invertebrates and lower vertebrates. For mammals use Helly's fluid.

Régaud's

3% potassium dichromate	80 ml
40% formaldehyde	20 ml

Régaud's is good for mitochondria, penetrating evenly and rapidly. Fix for 6–18 h. For Champy's fluid, replace the formaldehyde with 80 ml 1% chromic acid and 46 ml 2% osmium tetroxide. Champy's fluid is good for yolk, lipids and fatty tissues.

Elftman's fixative

Mercuric chloride	5 g
Potassium dichromate	2.5 g
Distilled water	to 100 ml

Fix for 3 days at room temperature. This is good for lipid preservation, especially in cryostat sections cut after fixation.

von Orth's fluid

Potassium dichromate	5.6 g
Sodium sulphate (anhydrous)	1.0 g
Distilled water	90 ml
40% formaldehyde	10 ml

Add the reagents in the order stated. This fixative must be freshly made; it will not keep. von Orth's is good for mitochondria and other cytoplasmic organelles.

Table 2.1: *continued*

Picric acid fixatives
Bouin's

Saturated aqueous picric acid (2%)	750 ml
40% formaldehyde	250 ml
Acetic acid	50 ml

This mixture keeps very well, and is useful as a field fixative. Fix for 6–24 h. Transfer the tissue directly to 70% alcohol. A micro-anatomical fixative which demonstrates kidney badly, but chromosomes and marine invertebrates well. Dilute by 1/2 or 1/3 for fixing embryos. It is not suited to tissues intended for frozen sectioning.

Allen's B-15

Bouin's fluid	100 ml
Chromic acid	1.5 g
Urea	2.0 g

Add the chromic acid to the Bouin's which has been heated to 37°C; stir, then add the urea. Once the urea is dissolved, cool slowly. This fixative is useful for plant tissue which is difficult to fix, such as plant buds. It must be made up fresh and used promptly before it goes green. Small blocks are fixed for 1 h; larger blocks for 4 h–overnight. A very prolonged wash in 70% alcohol over 2 days is needed to wash out all the picric acid.

Gendre's fluid

Saturated picric acid (9%) in 95% ethanol	200 ml
40% formaldehyde	37.5 ml
Acetic acid (glacial)	12.5 ml

Fix animal tissues for 1–4 h. Very similar to Rossman's (10% formalin in saturated picric acid in absolute ethanol). Both are good for glycogen preservation in liver.

Acetic acid fixatives
Carnoy's

Absolute ethyl alcohol	60 ml
Chloroform	30 ml
Acetic acid (glacial)	10 ml

A very rapidly penetrating fixative, which causes much shrinkage. It is useful for urgent biopsies, smears, intracellular glycogen and for chromosomes, which are well preserved. Fix small blocks, no thicker than 3 mm, for 1 h and transfer to 95% alcohol without washing. Carnoy's cannot be used with cellulose (e.g. Millipore) filters where these have been used as a substrate to grow cultured cells. The acetic acid can be reduced to 5%. In plant histology, Carnoy's can be used for up to 10 min to fix downy, resinous or impervious structures before secondary fixation in CRAF.

Carnoy–Lebrun's

Absolute ethyl alcohol	20 ml
Chloroform	20 ml
Acetic acid (glacial)	20 ml
Mercuric chloride to saturation	6 g

Not for routine use, but a very rapid botanical fixative. Fix for up to 30 min. It causes much shrinkage.

Table 2.1: *continued*

Methacarn

Methanol	60 ml
Chloroform	30 ml
Acetic acid (glacial)	10 ml

Fix tissue which is no more than 3 cm thick for 18–24 h, or up to 3 days if needed. This fixative is ideal for phase-partition studies. To prevent excessive shrinkage, tissues should not be rinsed in water or allowed to dry out. Process tissues by the routine given in the reference. It is good for studying fibrous proteins. Devised by Puchtler *et al.* (1970).

Clarke's

Absolute alcohol	75 ml
Acetic acid (glacial)	25 ml

This rapidly penetrating fixative gives good nuclear fixation, and is best suited to fixing smears, tissue-culture monolayers of cells and chromosome preparations. Fix for 12–24 h, although much shorter periods can suffice where speed is essential. Wash in 70% alcohol.

Newcomer's fixative

Isopropanol (propan-2-ol)	60 ml
Propionic acid	30 ml
Diethyl-ether	10 ml
Acetone	10 ml
Dioxan	10 ml

This is a very rapid penetrator and so causes excessive shrinkage, but it is good for chromatin and mucopolysaccharides. Tissue blocks should be small (no larger than 3 mm^3); fix these for 12–18 h at 40°C. Smaller blocks (up to 3 mm thick) should be fixed for 2–3 h. It is preferred to Carnoy's by some workers.

Cytological fixatives (see also Chapter 5)

Böhm–Sprenger's

Methanol	85 ml
40% formaldehyde	10 ml
Acetic acid (glacial)	5 ml

Fix tissue blocks for 3–8 h, and smears for 30–60 min at room temperature. Gross shrinkage and loss of lipids is apparent.

Ether-alcohol

70% ethanol	50 ml
Diethyl-ether	50 ml

A very rapid, but extremely flammable, fixative for smears. Exercise great *care* in use.

Schaudinn's

Mercuric chloride (sat. aqueous—8%)	50 ml
Absolute ethanol	25 ml

This was advocated by Giemsa for smears, particularly those likely to detach from the slide. Tissues, however, are shrunk extensively. Wet-fix smears for 10–20 min.

2.8 Secondary fixation

Tissues fixed in formalin mixtures are able to be fixed by more powerful subsequent mixtures, particularly mercuric chloride, Helly's fluid and Flemming's fluid. Some workers post-fix with 3% potassium dichromate to demonstrate mitochondria or myelin. Tissue blocks are left for 7 days, sections for 12–24 h, and small gross specimens overnight in the dichromate solution, which is followed by a wash for at least 30 min in running water. Tandler (1990) reports using standard electron microscopical aldehyde fixatives for a few minutes followed by fixation in phosphate-buffered 10% formalin, or other light microscopical fixative. The advantages claimed for this type of secondary fixation are that large blocks can be processed for combined light/electron microscope studies, that plastic embedding need not restrict the range of stains used, and finally that cytological detail of double-fixed material is superior to that which has been conventionally fixed.

2.9 Preservatives

There are few preservatives which will allow subsequent microscopical study, and suggestions are given in *Table 2.2*. Some, such as Kaiserling III, are based on glycerol, and are often recommended for museum specimens (Daws, 1990). Blaydes' formula is quoted for preserving the green colour in plants (Blaydes, 1937). Formalin should not be buffered to neutrality where it is to be used in a simple preparation, as precipitates may form in the cell. The two simplest preservatives are 70% alcohol with the addition of a little glycerol and thymol (to inhibit evaporation and the growth of moulds) or weak (5%) formol-saline in 0.85% sodium chloride. Thymol may cause deposits, or some stains to fade; alternatives are 1% propylene phenoxetol and 0.1% *p*-chlorophenoxetol.

2.10 Washing tissues

Tissues that must have the fixative washed out before subsequent processing (to avoid the deposition of insoluble protein precipitates) can be treated with the three siphon washers shown in *Figure 2.2*. These are more effective than a stream of tap water, especially if the inlet tube does not reach to the bottom of the washing vessel. Where this is the case, a layer of fixative mixture may remain at the bottom of the vessel to bathe the

Table 2.2:   List of different preservatives

Blaydes' [a]	
95% ethanol	45 ml
40% formaldehyde	5 ml
Acetic acid (glacial)	5 ml
Copper (II) sulphate	0.2 g
Distilled water	45 ml
Gatenby and Painter's [b]	
95% ethanol	25 ml
Glycerol	25 ml
Distilled water	50 ml
Amman's lacto-phenol [c]	
Lactic acid	20 g
Glycerol	34 ml
Phenol	20 g
Distilled water	20 ml

[a] Merely the addition of copper (II) sulphate to FAA fixative, often used for botanical tissues. The copper (II) sulphate will help preserve the green colour of plants. Gray (1954) recommends adding 1% ferric ammonium sulphate where haematoxylin staining follows.
[b] Useful for plant tissues.
[c] Can also be used as a fixative. Dissolve the phenol completely in the water and add the lactic acid and then glycerol. Reduce the glycerol to 17 ml for fungal hyphae, and 8 ml for general mycology. Aniline blue WS, acid fuchsin and Fast green FCF can all be added at 0.5% to give a staining fixative. The mixture can also be used to clear sections and small whole mounts and is a useful temporary mountant of high refractive index. Keep the mixture in a dark glass bottle; it is corrosive, and dissolves varnish. Seal using glycerol jelly and gold-size before finally ringing.

blocks while the water is replaced above them. Where washing will either cause swelling of the tissues (e.g. washing after picric acid will cause collagen to swell) or is not required for removing fixative constituents, tissues may be transferred to ethyl alcohol for subsequent processing. Very fine suspensions can be washed either by centrifugation and resuspension, or by placing the sample in an inclined trough within a sink under a constant slow-flowing stream of water. *Table 2.3* gives the various washing routines recommended after each fixation procedure.

2.11 Microwaves in histology

The use of microwaves in biology for improving and shortening both fixation and staining of tissue is a rapidly growing practice. For reproducible results the temperature rise must be defined and strictly controlled. Providing that either the tissue can withstand the temperature applied, or that the temperature in the microwave can be adequately

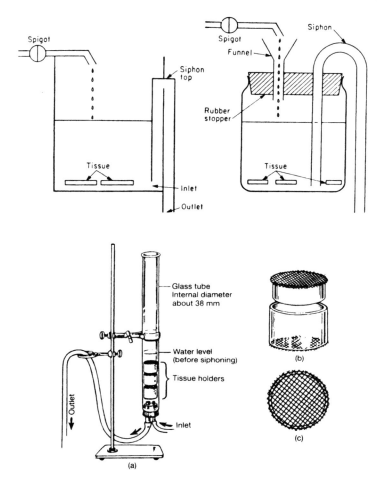

Figure 2.2: Siphonage tissue washers. Top: two models recommended by Lillie and Fullmer (1976) *Histopathological Technic and Practical Histochemistry*, 4th edn, reproduced with permission from McGraw-Hill. Bottom: design of Tolles and Newcomber (1950) *Stain Technol.* **25**, 23–24, redrawn in Davenport (1960) *Histological and Histochemical Technics*, reproduced with permission from Williams & Wilkins and Saunders College Publishing, respectively. (a) Assembled apparatus; (b) tissue holder; (c) bottom view of tissue holder.

controlled, microwave methods are superior to conventional methods of fixing and staining tissues (Jackson, 1990; van de Kant *et al.*, 1990; Kok and Boon, 1990) and are useful in preventing extraction of soluble lipids and proteins.

Water has a particularly high dipole moment when heated with microwaves of 2.45 GHz giving a large temperature rise quickly and evenly compared to convection heating methods. A molecule with a dipole moment of zero is not influenced by microwaves, which pass through at the speed of light without discharging energy to the material. In addition to the dipole moment it is important to know the penetration depth of micro-

Table 2.3: List of treatment routines for different groups of fixatives

Wash in running water 12–24 h:	*Transfer to 85% ethanol*
Champy's	B-5
Flemming's	Formol-sublimate
Helly's (Zenker-formol)	
Lewitsky–Baker's	*Transfer to 95% ethanol*
Navashin's	Carnoy's
Newcomer's	Carnoy–Lebrun's
von Orth's	Heidenhein's SUSA
Sanfelice's	Rossman's
Régaud's	
Zenker's	
Transfer to 50% ethanol	*Transfer to ethanol*
FAA	Clarke's
Glutaraldehyde	Ether-alcohol (same strength as fixative)
Schaudinn's	Gendre's
Transfer to 70% ethanol	*Transfer to absolute methanol*
Allen's B-15	Methacarn
Bouin's	
Randolph's CRAF	
Formalin-alcohol	
10% buffered formalin	
Formalin	
10% Formol-saline	
10% Formol-calcium	
10% Formol-sucrose	

waves through a substance. In a vacuum the microwavelength is about 12.2 cm, while in water it is 1.4 cm. Penetration depth is inversely proportional to electrical conductivity: ice is 'transparent', but microwaves penetrate metals poorly. Human tissues are penetrable for about 2 cm; domestic aluminium foil (ca. 25 μm thick) is penetrated only 1–2 μm by microwaves and so is an effective shield. Tissue biopsies or sections should not exceed twice the penetration depth for even heating. Microwaving will cause some shrinkage, but not usually as much as chemical fixing and processing.

2.12 Microwaving formalin-fixed tissues

Boon *et al.* (1988) recommend using 10% 0.1 M phosphate-buffered formalin pH 7.4 of 227 mOsm to fix tissues. Superior results are obtained after immersion for 4 h in formalin, rather than microwaving fresh tissue in fixative. Microwaving is then carried out for 1.5 min at 700 W, to achieve a temperature rise of 50–60°C. Since most of the formalin is present as methylene glycol, microwaving does four things: (a) the slow reaction of formalin within the tissue is enhanced, hence (b) more methylene glycol dissociates to replace it, (c) the methylene glycol is prevented from poly-merizing and (d) the formaldehyde-fixed tissue then forms a barrier to further penetration of fixative.

Some tissue, notably neural or lymphoid tissue, does not respond well to microwaving. Low heat levels or reduced heating times can cause perinuclear halos as membranes separate, while excessive heating causes poor preservation and vacuolation. Nuclei are rendered more prominent by microwaves, and lung tissue benefits from heating to 77°C since air expansion at this temperature counteracts tissue collapse at lower temperatures, or during conventional processing.

The major barrier to widespread use of microwaves for preparing specimens is reproducibility. Most domestic ovens are too primitive to ensure adequate heating. Each microwave oven has its own characteristic 'hot' and 'cold' spots, which can be critical when trying to accurately heat tissues of small surface area. In addition, the field intensity in the micro-wave oven will change when it is filled depending upon the vapour pressure, thermic and dipole moment of the treated tissue. Curved con-tainers can act as 'lenses' focusing the microwaves and producing hot spots. This is why eggs (at the critical diameter of refraction of 4 cm) explode readily when microwaved! Therefore, the best containers for even heating are rectangular. An even heat distribution may be achieved using a turntable, stirrers, power cycling, and blowing air through heated fluids. The best load position for an individual microwave must be determined by experiment.

Temperature measurement inside microwave ovens is not straight-forward. Fluid-filled thermometers cannot be used because of the high risk of explosion. Fibre-optic thermometers are expensive, and thermocouples can be prone to over-registering temperature, especially when a poor absorber of microwaves is being heated. Furthermore, a microwave is either switched on or off; intermediate heating levels are determined by cycling between on and off, and cycle times will vary between different ovens. It is necessary to plot heating versus cycle time calibration curves in order to determine for how long to microwave reagents in each case. Accurate heating is more likely to be achieved where cycle times are short, and small volumes of fluid avoided, so that individual energy bursts do not cause too large fluctuations. Because of all these potential variables, procedures for specific tissues must be worked out empirically in each case, and solutions should initially be heated slowly to avoid boiling or altering their characteristics.

Paraffin is almost transparent to microwaves, making it difficult to keep the temperature of the tissue constant at 67°C optimum. To overcome this ovens fitted with a temperature probe or constant heat setting are required for reproducible work. The Miele M696 and H2500 (Energy Beam Sciences) are two such examples. Materials should be put into suitable microwave plastic containers or cuvettes, and not into glass which can absorb microwaves to different extents. Although propan-2-ol (isopro-panol) diffuses out of tissues slowly in conventional processing, it has a high dipole moment and boils at a lower temperature than xylene. Propan-2-ol is therefore excellent for microwaving, completes the dehydration series and can effectively be boiled off from a paraffin section at 67°C.

2.12.1 Leiden fixative

This fixative is similar to the commercially available Kryofix® and tissues can apparently be stored in it for long periods of time. The molecular weight of the polyethylene glycol (PEG) is lower than that used for cytological fixation, to allow rapid diffusion into the tissues.

96% alcohol	500 ml
Distilled water	430 ml
PEG 300	70 ml

The biopsies are removed from the fixative and placed in $2 \times 2 \times 0.5$ cm plastic tissue cassettes with lids in a rack in absolute ethanol held in a plastic container. Specimens received in 10% formalin are placed into 70% alcohol prior to treatment in absolute alcohol. The tissue is then micro-waved in propan-2-ol and the cassette holding rack is changed. The specimens are then microwaved in Paramat wax at 67°C and 82°C, and then vacuum embedded in the routine way (Section 3.5).

2.13 Microwaving paraffin sections

Three methods have been published by Kok *et al.* (1988) for microwaving and paraffin embedding of different-sized tissues. Although propan-2-ol is cited as being more suitable than xylene, the latter can be used in the protocols if an extra 5 min microwaving is allowed, and the first paraffin bath is heated slowly. Unlike propan-2-ol, xylene is not as equally micro-waveable as paraffin, and unless the first paraffin bath is heated slowly, pockets of xylene remaining in the tissue can rise in temperature much more quickly than intended and boil off violently, disrupting tissue.

2.14 Microwaving cryostat sections

Conventionally processed cryostat sections never give such a crisp result as paraffin- or resin-embedded material. However, if the initial freezing step is carried out rapidly to avoid ice crystal artifact, and if the sections are fixed and microwaved within 15 sec of cutting, then consistently good results are possible with particularly sharp nuclear structure. Ideally, the microwave oven should be placed next to the cryostat. The sections are

picked up singly on a warm slide, covered with a few drops of Kryofix®
and microwaved on top of a polystyrene (microwave transparent) platform
for about 20 sec at 450 W.

2.15 Staining reactions

Because most dyestuffs diffuse into tissues, microwaving can speed up
staining reactions considerably. Care is needed in deciding upon exact
protocols, since microwaving can also increase the risk of artifacts and
tissue loss. Sections may be mounted onto 0.25% gelatin-coated slides
without erroneous results. Metallic staining, in particular, benefits from
microwaving with considerable time saving (Hopwood, 1992). Dye–substrate binding interactions are enhanced by microwaving, with more
intense results and less background (Barone, 1993; Suurmeijer et al.,
1990). Details of immunocytochemical staining are given in Boon et al.
(1990) and Shi et al. (1991); a comparative study between microwaves and
enzymes for unmasking antigens has recently been carried out by Cattoretti et al. (1993).

Safety

Do not heat paper or metal foil in a microwave—these can spark or ignite
and damage the oven. Sparks can also result from pencil graphite used on
frosted microscope slides, and a diamond or spirit pen should be used
instead. Formalin fixation can be enhanced by microwaving, but formaldehyde is volatile, and should therefore be microwaved in a fume hood.

References

Baker JR. (1950) *Cytological Technique.* Methuen, London.
Barone CA. (1993) Microwave stimulation for commonly-used mordants. *Biotechnic Histochem.*, **68**, 122–124.
Blaydes GW. (1937) Preserving natural colour in green plants. *Science* **85**, 126–127.
Boon ME, Gerrits PO, Moorlag HE, Nieuwenhuis P, Kok LP. (1988) Formaldehyde
fixation and microwave irradiation. *Histochem. J.* **20**, 313–322.
Boon ME, Hendrikse FCJ, Kok PG, Bolhuis P, Kok LP. (1990) A practical approach to
routine immunostaining of paraffin sections in the microwave oven. *Histochem. J.* **22**,
347–352.

Cattoretti G, Pileri S, Parravicini C, Becker MHG, Poggi S, Bifulco C, Key G, D'Amato L, Sabattini E, Feudale E, Reynolds F, Gerdes J, Rilke F. (1993) Antigen unmasking on formalin-fixed, paraffin-embedded tissue sections. *J. Pathol.* **171**, 83–98.

Chayen J, Bitensky L. (1991) *Practical Histochemistry*, 2nd edn. John Wiley & Sons, Chichester.

Côté SL, Ribiero-da-Silva A, Cuello AC. (1993) Current protocols for light microscopic immunocytochemistry. In *Immunochemistry II.* (ed. AC Cuello) John Wiley & Sons, Chichester, pp. 147–168.

Crawford GNC, Barer R. (1951) The action of formaldehyde on living cells as studied by phase-contrast microscopy. *Q. J. Microscop. Sci.* **92**, 403–452.

Culling CFA, Allison RT, Barr WT. (1985) *Cellular Pathology Technique*, 4th edn. Butterworths, London.

Dapson RW. (1993) Fixation for the 1990's: a review of needs and accomplishments. *Biotechnic Histochem.* **68**, 75–82.

Daws JJ. (1990) Museum and other demonstration techniques. In *Theory and Practice of Histological Techniques*, 3rd edn (eds JD Bancroft and A Stevens). Churchill Livingstone, Edinburgh, pp. 667–687.

Drury RAB, Wallington EA. (1980) *Carleton's Histological Technique*, 5th edn. Oxford University Press, Oxford.

Fox CH, Johnson FB, Whiting J, Roller PP. (1985) Formaldehyde fixation. *J. Histochem. Cytochem.* **33**, 845–853.

Gray P. (1954) *The Microtomist's Formulary and Guide.* Blakiston, New York.

Harvey DMR. (1982) Freeze-substitution. *J. Microsc.* **127**, 209–221.

Hayat MA. (1989) *Principles and Techniques of Electron Microscopy: Biological Applications*, 3rd edn. Macmillan, Basingstoke.

Hopwood D. (1985) Cell and tissue fixation 1972–1982. *Histochem. J.* **17**, 389–442.

Hopwood D. (1990) Fixation and Fixatives. In *Theory and Practice of Histological Techniques*, 3rd edn (eds JD Bancroft and A Stevens). Churchill Livingstone, Edinburgh, pp. 21–42.

Hopwood D, Slidders W, Yeaman GR. (1989) Tissue fixation with phenol-formaldehyde for routine histopathology. *Histochem. J.* **21**, 228–234.

Hopwood D. (1992) Microwaves in tissue preparation. *Proc. R. Microscop. Soc.* **27**, 71–74.

Horobin RW. (1982) *Histochemistry: an Explanatory Outline of Histochemistry and Biophysical Staining.* Gustav Fischer Verlag, Stuttgart; Butterworths, London.

Howard WB, Willhite CC, Smart RA. (1989) Fixative evaluation and histologic appearance of embryonic rodent tissue. *Stain Technol.* **64**, 1–8.

Jackson P. (1990) Application of microwaves in biological specimen preparation. *Microsc. Anal.* **15**, 7–9.

Johnson WD, Lang CM, Johnson MT. (1978) Fixatives and methods of fixation in selected tissues of the Laboratory Rat. *Clin. Toxicol.* **12**, 583–600.

van de Kant HJG, de Rooij DG, Boon ME. (1990) Microwave stabilization versus chemical fixation. A morphometric study in glycolmethacrylate- and paraffin-embedded tissue. *Histochem. J.* **22**, 335–340.

Kiernan JA. (1990) *Histological & Histochemical Methods: Theory & Practice*, 2nd edn. Pergamon Press, Oxford.

Kok LP, Boon ME. (1990) Microwaves for microscopy. *J. Microsc.* **158**, 291–322.

Kok LP, Visser PE, Boon ME. (1988) Histoprocessing with the microwave oven: an update. *Histochem. J.* **20**, 323–328.

Leitch AR, Schwarzacher T, Jackson D, Leitch IJ. (1994) *In Situ Hybridization.* Royal Microscopical Society Handbook No. 27, BIOS Scientific Publishers, Oxford.

Lillie RD, Fullmer HM. (1976) *Histopathological Technique and Practical Histochemistry*, 4th edn. McGraw-Hill, New York.

Lillie RD, Pizzolato P, Vacca LL. (1973) Salt-Zenker, a stable, nonhaemolytic, formaldehyde-free fixative. *Am. J. Clin. Pathol.* **59**, 374–375

McLean IW, Nakane PK. (1974) Periodate-lysine-paraformaldehyde fixative, a new fixative for immunoelectron microscopy. *J. Histochem. Cytochem.* **22**, 1077–1083.

Maser MD, Powell III TE, Philpott CW. (1967) Relationships among pH, osmolality and concentration of fixative solutions. *Stain Technol.* **42**, 175–182.

Murray GI, Ewen SWB. (1991) A novel method for optimum biopsy specimen preservation for histochemical & immunohistochemical analysis. *Am. J. Clin. Pathol.* **95**, 131–136.

Nettleton GS, McAuliffe WG. (1986) A histological comparison of phase-partition fixation with fixation in aqueous solutions. *J. Histochem. Cytochem.* **34**, 795–800.

Pearse AGE. (1980) *Histochemistry: Theoretical and Applied*, Vol. 1, 4th edn. Churchill Livingstone, Edinburgh.

Pentilla A, McDowell ME, Trump BF. (1975) Effects of fixation and post-fixation treatments on volume of injured cells. *J. Histochem. Cytochem.* **22**, 251–270.

Puchtler H, Waldrop FS, Meloan SN, Terry MS, Conner HM. (1970) Methacarn (methanol-Carnoy) fixation. *Histochemie* **21**, 97–116.

Robinson DG, Ehlers U, Herken R, Hermann B, Mayer F, Schürmann F-W. (1987) *Methods of Preparation for Electron Microscopy*. Springer-Verlag, Berlin.

Ross BD. (1972) *Perfusion Techniques in Biochemistry*. Clarendon, Oxford.

Rostgaard J, Qvortrup K, Poulsen SS. (1993) Improvements in the technique of vascular perfusion-fixation employing a fluorocarbon-containing perfusate and a peristaltic pump controlled by pressure feedback. *J. Microsc.* **172**, 137–151.

Sato Y, Mukai K, Watanabe S, Goto M, Shimosato Y. (1986) The AMeX method. *Am. J. Pathol.* **125**, 431–435.

Shi S-R, Key ME, Kalra KI. (1991) Antigen retrieval in formalin-fixed, paraffin-embedded tissues: an enhancement method for immunohistochemical staining based on microwave oven heating of tissue sections. *J. Histochem. Cytochem.* **39**, 741–748.

Sims DE, Westfall JA, Kiorpes AL, Horne MM. (1991) Preservation of tracheal mucus by nonaqueous fixative. *Biotechnic Histochem.* **66**, 173–180.

Stahl WL, Baskin DG. (1993) Workshop on *in situ* hybridisation: what you need to know to get it to work. *J. Histochem. Cytochem.* **41**, 1721–1723.

Stickland NC. (1975) A Detailed analysis of the effects of various fixatives on animal tissues with particular reference to muscle tissue. *Stain Technol.* **50**, 255–264.

Suurmeijer AJH, Boon ME, Kok LP. (1990) Notes on the application of microwaves in histopathology. *Histochem. J.* **22**, 341–346.

Tandler B. (1990) Improved sectionability of paraffin-embedded specimens that initially are fixed in EM fixatives. *J. Electron Microsc. Tech.* **14**, 287–288.

Uehara F, Ohba N, Nakashima Y, Yanagita T, Ozawa M, Muramatsu T. (1993) A fixative suitable for *in situ* hybridization histochemistry. *J. Histochem. Cytochem.* **41**, 947–953.

Wilcox JN. (1993) Fundamental principles of *in situ* hybridization. *J. Histochem. Cytochem.* **41**, 1725–1733.

Wood RL, Luft JH. (1965) The influence of buffer systems on fixation with osmium tetroxide. *J. Ultrastruct. Res.* **12**, 22–45.

3   Tissue Processing

After fixation, the tissue must be processed for sectioning, staining and mounting. The flow chart in *Figure 3.1* shows some of the more common protocols used in tissue processing. In the simplest case the tissue is washed free of fixative, stained and mounted in an aqueous mountant. There is then no need to alternate between different processing phases unless the tissue has to be supported for microtomy, stained and mounted in a resinous medium—which is usually the case. The most common embedding media used to infiltrate specimens for microtomy are as follows.

(i)   Paraffin wax, or a variant such as PEG or ester wax.
(ii)   Water (as tissue water or aqueous medium) for frozen sections.
(iii)   Plastic resins.
(iv)   Celloidin or low viscosity nitrocellulose (LVN).

Since water is immiscible with most embedding media and mountants, and yet is the favoured diluent for most stains, tissues must be exchanged between these polar and organic reagents via a series of dehydrating and transition media. Most mountants and molten or hot paraffin wax are miscible with transition agents, but not with alcohols or water. The transition medium, therefore, serves to transfer the specimen from the dehydrating alcohol to the embedding medium and, later, the mountant. The times given in the schedules refer to animal tissues; plants composed of tougher tissues require correspondingly longer in all reagents. Generally, plant tissues should remain immersed for 8–12 h, and up to 24 h for very resistant or lignified tissues. Furthermore, the change between dehydrant and transition medium can be carried out stepwise (e.g. in the ratios 3:1; 1:1; 1:3) with 2–4 h at each step. If required, tough, woody tissues can be macerated (Section 5.6.1) before further processing.

The established name for the transition or ante-medium is 'clearing agent', since the most frequently used of these have the effect of rendering the tissues or sections almost clear on impregnation by raising the refractive index to approximately that of glass (RI = 1.52). It is incorrect to think that stained tissues necessarily become physically clear as they are passed from alcohol to the clearing medium, such as xylene—in fact, because xylene is very intolerant of any water, any incompletely dehydrated

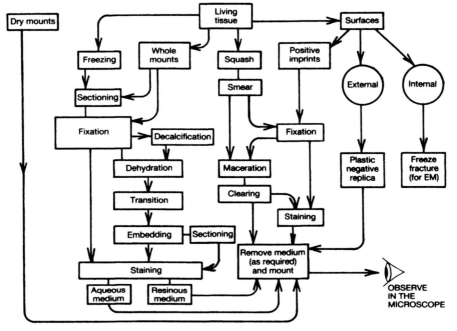

Figure 3.1:   Tissue processing. Flow chart showing the means, described in this chapter, by which tissues may be processed.

sections will be far from clear once they have passed through this transition medium!

It is important that tissues are thoroughly processed, for, although shrinkage and hardening are inevitable (see *Figure 4.19*), badly processed tissue cannot be adequately sectioned or prepared. All specimens should be reliably identified; the best way to do this is either to enclose them in purpose-made plastic cassettes, which can be written on with a soft (2B) pencil, or to include a hand-written paper label with the specimen through all the processing stages until the final embedding and blocking out. Do not use ink, for this will run, and either become illegible and/or contaminate processing fluids and tissue.

For hand-processing, wide-mouthed screw-topped or glass-stoppered jars are better suited than corked tubes, and the volume should be 20–50 times that of the specimen. Where a large number of specimens is automatically processed, plastic cassettes with plastic or metal lids are used. The tissue is eventually blocked out in the cassette: the lid is removed (to be reused if of metal) and the standard cassette used to form the base of the wax block which clamps into the microtome. Small specimens, which may be liable to pass through the mesh of the cassette, should be wrapped in lint-free coarse-weave bandage. Keep large tissues flat between cheesecloth held in a former (e.g. a small embroidery hoop).

It is of crucial importance for adequate processing that the blocks of tissue are cut small enough such that they move freely within the cassette and are not compressed. It is equally important that the tissues are agitated regularly throughout the schedule to assist diffusion and replacement of the processing fluids within the tissues. Incomplete dehydration causes undue shrinkage and hardening of tissues, and results in poor sections. Ethanol is a poor dehydrant in those tissues where it has been used as the fixative.

3.1 Dehydration

Most tissues are taken through a series of ethyl alcohol gradients from one bath or tank to another, either by hand or automatically (e.g. Roberts and Warren, 1987). In general, the time required to process tissues for sectioning will depend on the size of the least dimension of the tissue block. Most sequences start with 70% ethanol, although 50% or even 30% may be advocated for very delicate (e.g. embryonic) tissues. Ethyl alcohol is sold as absolute alcohol or as industrial methylated spirits (IMS). The latter has an added quantity of methanol to render it unfit for consumption, and IMS is considerably cheaper than absolute alcohol because it is not liable for Excise Duty. 74° over-proof IMS is equivalent to 99% ethanol; for an explanation of the relationship between proof and spirit strength, the reader is referred to the footnote on p. 56 of Culling *et al.* (1985). Provided that the last alcohol is changed frequently, it is not necessary to dry the alcohol with a molecular sieve or copper (II) sulphate unless embedding the tissue in a hydrophobic resin. Where these chemicals are used to dry the alcohol, ensure that layers of filter paper prevent particles of drying agent from contaminating the sample when the alcohol is drawn off.

For dehydration isopropanol (propan-2-ol) does not harden tissue to the same extent as ethanol. Acetone is good for rapid dehydration, but will cause extensive lipid loss and result in brittle as well as hard tissues. Other dehydrants are *n*-butyl alcohol (butan-1-ol), pyridine, PEG, and glycerol. Butan-1-ol is only partly miscible with water, but fully miscible with ethanol and transition media. It is useful where sections are blotted, extracting less stain than ethanol, but cannot be used with nitrocellulose, which is insoluble in butan-1-ol (Hemenway, 1930; Lang, 1937).

Dehydration will leach out lipids. The faster the transfer of material through the dehydration series, the less will this effect be. Dehydration at 4°C will also help retain lipids within tissues. Acetone extracts more lipid than ethanol, but it is employed because certain plastics (notably epoxy resins) are miscible with acetone obviating the need for a transition medium. An alternative, which may work where tissues respond badly to physical replacement of water, is chemical dehydration (Postek,

1978) using 2,2-dimethoxy-propane (DMP, acetone dimethylacetal). Some resins, notably LR White and LR Gold (Section 3.18.3) are intolerant of acetone, and should not be used following dehydration by acetone or DMP.

3.2 Transition media

Xylene (xylol, dimethylbenzene) is the most commonly used transition medium, both for embedding into and removing wax from sections and for mounting specimens into resin after dehydrating and staining. It is rapid in its action, and blocks up to 3 mm thick can be treated in as little as 20 min. Prolonged exposure can make soft tissues (e.g. brain and spleen) rather brittle, and xylene hardens tissue more than any other transition medium. Generally, those transition media with low viscosity and boiling points are removed most rapidly from wax, although chloroform is an exception. As a rule, the minimum exposure to the transition medium should be aimed for.

Benzene, carbon tetrachloride (tetrachloromethane) and chloroform (trichloromethane) have been used in the past as transition media, and although they harden tissue much less than xylene, they are highly toxic and carcinogenic, and nowadays are rarely used. Tissues that have been fixed in Clarke's, Methacarn or Carnoy's fluid should be hand-processed through chloroform. Tissue from Clarke's or Carnoy's fluid is passed through an equal mixture of ethanol and chloroform for 30–60 min followed by two changes of chloroform for the same length of time. Tissues fixed in Methacarn may be taken directly through two changes of chloroform for 30–60 min. Chloroform acts more slowly than xylene, is not flammable and does not harden tissue to the same extent. Furthermore, chloroform leaves tissue opaque rather than transparent, and tissues do not sink once impregnated; therefore, it must be used over a longer period of time to ensure complete transition. Chloroform must be completely removed for good quality sectioning, and should not be heated.

Toluene (toluol, methylbenzene) and cedarwood oil are popular transition media for delicate tissues because they do not render the tissue as brittle as xylene, and cedarwood oil does not cause as much shrinkage. They are both slower acting than xylene and tissues should remain immersed until they have sunk to the bottom of the container. Tissue blocks of 2–8 mm across the smallest face (see Section 2.2.1) must remain immersed for 3–5 days. Smaller blocks (1 mm^3) can be left one entire day and night with a single change half-way through.

To obviate changing tissues from the last alcohol into cedarwood oil at an inconvenient time, a phase-partition system can be used. The container is half-filled with cedarwood oil, and the lighter phase of alcohol layered on top. The tissue is carefully immersed in the alcohol, where it will initially lie at the phase interface and gradually sink into the oil. A fresh change of oil must be used prior to embedding into wax. Cedarwood oil is also very useful for clearing tough or heterogenous tissues (skin, uterus, muscle) which are difficult to cut, because it improves their consistency for sectioning. Tissues can be left in cedarwood oil for several months without harm, and can remain in the tissues to some extent without impairing the sectioning quality. However, the slightest trace of oil left in the tissues at the embedding step will soften the wax to such an extent that sections are impossible or difficult to cut. For this reason, some workers advocate a short (1 h) transfer to toluene or xylene prior to infiltration with wax.

Other little-used transition media include the essential oils terpineol, benzyl and methyl benzoate, isoamyl acetate, methyl salicylate and clove oil. Methyl salicylate, terpineol, cedarwood and clove oil are useful as clearing agents where the purity of the absolute alcohol cannot be guaranteed, since they have a relatively high tolerance for water. Aniline oil, bergamot oil and terpineol will tolerate about 10%, cedarwood oil 5% water, but xylene only 1% residual water. Akin to the essential oils are the citrus fruit oils (e.g. Histoclear®) derived from food stuffs. Excellent for initial processing, they should be used with caution when finally mounting sections after staining, as their acid nature can cause dyes to leach out and/or fade with time. Dioxan (Guyer, 1953) has the advantage that it is freely miscible with water, ethanol and paraffin wax.

3.3 Processing schedules

It is generally not wise to use a rapid processing schedule. Where this is imperative, cut frozen tissue, which is the most rapid procedure, or treat as below. Rapid embedding using resins is not recommended. For rapid wax embedding, blocks should not be more than 3 mm thick.

A rapid processing schedule for tissues
1. Fix in Carnoy's fluid   30–60 min
2. Three changes of absolute alcohol   30 min each
3. Two changes of xylene   15 min each
4. Three changes of paraffin (under vacuum) 20 min each
5. Embed
Total time (including changeover times)   5 h

The process may be hastened using warm fixative (e.g. 10% formalin at 60°C), or otherwise an alcoholic fixative, starting the dehydration with 90% alcohol or using acetone, followed by xylene as the transition medium and impregnating with wax under vacuum at all stages (see also Brain, 1974).

Although automatic schedules are convenient, manual schedules may not only be faster, but can be adapted to take account of very large or small pieces of tissue, or allow the use of very volatile or flammable fluids which would otherwise be too hazardous to use on an automatic processor. A general schedule, over 3 nights and 2 days for blocks up to 5 mm thick is as follows.

A manual processing schedule

1.	10% formalin	Overnight	17.00–08.30
2.	70% ethanol	2 h	08.30–10.30
3.	90% ethanol	2 h	10.30–12.30
4.	Absolute ethanol	1.5 h	12.30–14.00
5.	Absolute ethanol	1.5 h	14.00–15.30
6.	Absolute ethanol	1.5 h	15.30–17.00
7.	Absolute ethanol	Overnight	17.00–08.30
8.	Xylene	1.5 h	08.30–10.00
9.	Xylene	2 h	10.00–12.00
10.	Paraffin wax	2.5 h	12.00–14.30
11.	Paraffin wax	2.5 h	14.30–17.00
12.	Paraffin wax	Overnight	17.00–08.30

Other suitable processing schedules are given in Gordon (1990).

3.4 Automatic processing

Where specimens are prepared in large numbers, automatic processing has a distinct advantage over manual techniques, ensuring uniformity, reduced exposure to harmful reagents and saving of time. Various machines have been marketed; some of the older designs are still widely used (for illustrations see Drury and Wallington, 1980; Culling *et al.* 1985), but the enclosed type of processor is now increasingly popular, due to the Control of Substances Hazardous to Health (COSHH) and revised legal regulations. Two modern designs are illustrated in *Figure 3.2*.

Two schedules are given below. Schedule (A) will deliver processed tissue ready for embedding at the start of the next day, and allows for two or more baskets to follow each other. Schedule (B) allows a short overnight run, following tissue dissection and preparation in the afternoon, permitting embedding of the tissues prior to sectioning the following morning. The tissues should ideally be no more than 3 mm, and larger blocks should be fixed for longer before processing.

Automatic processing schedules

		(A)		(B)	
1.	10% formalin	2 h	09.00–11.00	1.5 h	16.00–17.30
2.	70% ethanol	2 h	11.00–13.00	30 min	17.30–18.00

3.	80% ethanol	2 h	13.00–15.00	1 h	18.00–19.00
4.	90% ethanol	2 h	15.00–17.00	1 h	19.00–20.00
5.	Absolute ethanol	2 h	17.00–19.00	1.5 h	20.00–21.30
6.	Absolute ethanol	2 h	19.00–21.00	1 h	21.30–22.30
7.	Absolute ethanol	2 h	21.00–23.00	1 h	22.30–23.30
8.	Absolute ethanol	2 h	23.00–01.00	30 min	23.30–00.00
9.	Xylene	2 h	01.00–03.00	2 h	00.00–02.00
10.	Xylene	2 h	03.00–05.00	2 h	02.00–04.00
11.	Paraffin wax	2 h	05.00–07.00	2 h	04.00–06.00
12.	Paraffin wax	2 h	07.00–09.00	2 h	06.00–08.00

Trichloroethane may be substituted for xylene on account of its lower toxicity and flammability. Gordon (1990) suggests two changes of 10% formalin, a single 75% intermediate dehydration step and five changes of absolute alcohol. Adequate formalin fixation is essential to prevent an alcohol fixation pattern emerging. It is advisable for larger blocks or tougher, less penetrable tissue (e.g. uterus, or those with much connective tissue) to be fixed as slices during the previous day in 10% formalin before taking blocks and starting the processing schedule. Where the processing must run over a weekend, times can be extended in the first alcohol and wax. A table of other processing schedules can be found in Lillie and Fullmer (1976).

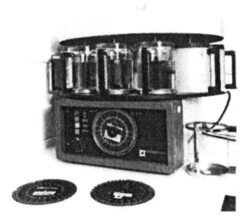
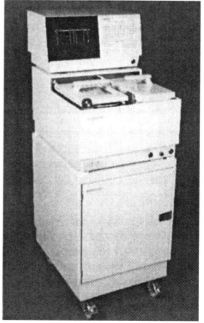

Figure 3.2: Automatic tissue processors. The Histokinette 2000 (photograph courtesy of Leica, left) and Hypercentre XP (photograph courtesy of Shandon, Life Sciences International, right) are examples of carousel and enclosed tissue processors. Two notched wheels, which regulate the programmes of the carousel, can be seen in the foreground.

3.5 Embedding media

Good sectioning requires specimens to be embedded in media of approximately equal density and resilience, so that adequate support is given, and the tissues do not separate under the force of sectioning. In addition, it is sometimes useful to use hydrophilic embedding media to avoid the use of transition agents before and after using aqueous stains. Several embedding media have been developed to meet the needs of biological workers. The most commonly used embedding medium is wax, but synthetic resins are increasingly being used.

The chosen method of embedding will depend not only upon the physical properties of the tissues being examined, but also on the intended thickness of the sections to be cut. Sectioning of material embedded in paraffin is best carried out in the range from 6–12 μm. Because of its manner of penetration, paraffin is best suited to tissues treated with coagulant fixatives. Since better cytological detail results from tissues fixed using non-coagulant fixatives and embedded in plastic, the continued use of paraffin on a wide scale is due to the ease and rapidity with which good sections can be cut, and the large number of staining methods that can be employed on paraffin-embedded tissue. Resin sections are superior where semi-thin sections are required to visualize cytological detail that would otherwise be obscured in a thicker wax section, or where the tissue is hard or must also be viewed by electron microscopy. Semi-thin resin sections are usually cut in the range 0.2–0.5 μm with a steel, tungsten carbide or glass knife.

3.5.1 Wax embedding

There are several ways in which paraffin blocks may be cast.
  (i)   Using re-useable metal or plastic moulds in an embedding centre.
  (ii) Using a disposable paper or metal foil mould.
  (iii) Using Leuckhart 'L' pieces.
  (iv) Using a watch glass for very small or delicate specimens.

Most routine laboratories use mild steel moulds for embedding large quantities of tissues up to 20 × 35 × 5 mm. A better block is cast from a shallow mould with a large surface area, than a deep one with a small surface area. Before any method of embedding, the tissue is removed from the processing cassette or container and inspected. From an examination of the appearance and texture of the block, it is possible to determine whether infiltration has taken place properly. Tissues should be rigid and covered with a coat of molten wax, and there should be no exposed unprocessed tissue.

Wax should be stored in an oven at about 2–3°C above its melting point. If the wax is kept too hot, it will oxidize forming a yellowish mixture and losing much of its crystal structure. Filter the molten wax into three metal jugs, and keep one for each wax change. Double-filter the last wax change, and let the wax stand well before it is needed so that air bubbles may escape from the mass. The final embedding is often done under vacuum, especially for tissues with large or numerous cavities, such as lung alveoli, which trap air. For routine purposes −500 mmHg is sufficient, but this value should be reduced by half for tissues of the central nervous system. Most tissues will withstand a partial vacuum as low as −535 mmHg. If a vacuum apparatus is used, the rubber sealing ring should ideally be unseated and removed after each use so that it does not perish *in situ.*

Small objects may be transferred using a heated pipette: score, remove the tip and flame the sharp edge. Otherwise, wide-bore tubing attached to a pipette bulb can also be used. A bent seeker can be useful whilst embedding to free a specimen that sets too quickly. Heat the seeker and pass it through the wax mass under the specimen to free any object which sets before complete orientation. Place the specimen eccentrically in the block, since the wax will solidify last in the central zone, producing looser and larger crystals which cut less well than the rest of the block.

For embedding, the wax should be double-filtered, poured at about 5–10°C above its melting point and, once the tissue is embedded, the block cooled rapidly. Do not plunge the block below the surface of the cooling water, as the weight of water may break the skin of the wax, or dissolve it if it is a water-soluble type. Rapid cooling is good, but too sudden cooling may cause any remaining air dissolved in the wax due to lack of or improper embedding (especially if there are large amounts) to come out of solution. Let the water come up to the top of the mould. The lip formed on the paper boat will allow the boat to float on the surface of the cooling water. While paper boats will flex to accommodate the considerable shrinking of the cooling wax, so obviating localized pressure regions, boats involve the use of much surplus wax. The maximum reasonable size for such blocks is about 40 × 20 × 20 mm.

To avoid the top layer of congealed wax being carried down with the object, where its differing crystal structure will impede sectioning, melt the top coat of wax with heated forceps or a small bunsen flame (the pilot light) just prior to embedding the object. Do not move the block unduly once the tissue is embedded until the wax is hardened throughout: this will avoid wax crystal movement, specimen damage and air bubble formation. Blow on the wax surface to cool it after embedding, and move the block carefully to the ice-water. Leave the block to cool evenly throughout before cutting, either in the refrigerator or at room temperature. Blocks may be stored in 5% glycerol in 70% alochol, but are usually stored in air. Wax should not have traces of clearing agent—although wax blocks will tolerate *very* small quantities of cedarwood oil. Blocks that exhibit streaks or white starry regions have been cast from polluted wax. The excess wax should be removed, and the object re-embedded through a series of fresh waxes.

An embedding centre holds the infiltrated specimens in a wax bath, delivers a supply of molten wax and has a cold stage for rapid cooling of the block. Remove the tissue, inspect it and determine the best orientation for casting. Fill a pressed steel mould of sufficient size such that there is about 2–3 mm wax around the tissue. Leave the meniscus slightly proud of the well; it will reduce on cooling. Insert and orientate the tissue quickly, and cool on the cold stage. Keep the block still for a minute or so until the wax has solidified. Modern embedding centres are shown in *Figure 3.3*; refer to the individual manufacturer's brochure for further details.

Prior to the introduction of the embedding centre, the traditional method was to fold a paper mould by hand (old glossy magazines are suitable), or on a block-former, and cast in this. Metal foil can also be used, and is a better heat conductor when cooling. Fold the material as shown in *Figure 3.4*. Wet the underside of the paper box and press it onto a metal plate. Pour in wax to three-quarters fill the mould. When the bottom layer has started to solidify, yet is still plastic, lift the specimen out of the final wax with seekers, forceps or a fine spatula and orientate it as desired.

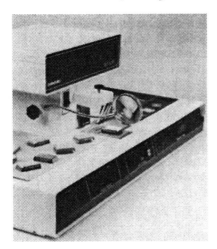

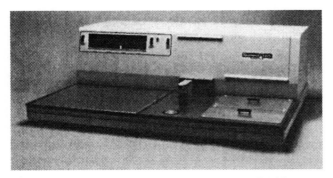

Figure 3.3: Automatic wax embedding centres. The Histocentre 2 (photography courtesy of Shandon, Life Sciences International, top) and Blockmaster III (photograph courtesy of Raymond A Lamb, bottom) are typical examples of wax embedding centres.

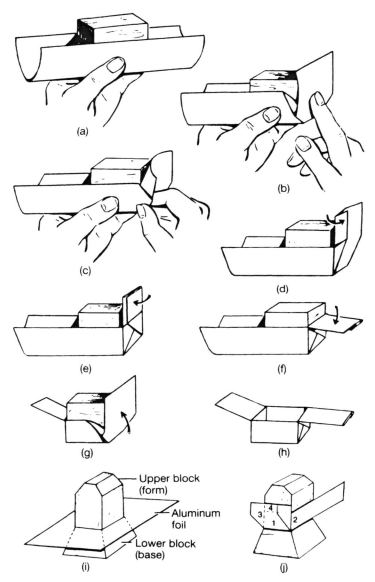

(a)

(b)

(c)

(d)

(e)

(f)

(g)

(h)

Upper block
(form)

Aluminum
foil

Lower block
(base)

(i)

(j)

Figure 3.4:   Preparation of moulds for casting wax blocks. A rectangular piece of paper is used and folded around a wooden former (a–h). The label can either be written on the extended tab or embedded (e.g. see *Figure 4.2*) when the final block is cast. (i) and (j) show how aluminium foil can be folded; the mould is formed around the upper block (folds 1–4) while the lower block aids handling. Reproduced from Davenport (1960) *Histological and Histochemical Technics* with permission from Saunders College Publishing.

Breathe on the surface of the wax to form a skin, and place it in a large container of ice-cold water. A quick method which suffices for small objects is to wrap masking tape around the base of an upturned McCartney bottle or cork. The depth of the block should not be more than the diameter of the block face, or slow cooling results.

Leuckhart pieces (see *Figure 4.5*) may also be used to cast blocks. They are also referred to as 'L' pieces, and are made of brass or steel. Leuckharts are used as a pair in conjunction with a metal or glass baseplate. Before use, the plate and the 'L' pieces should be cooled and smeared with a thin layer of grease, albumen or glycerol to assist in releasing the block without fracturing it. Arrange the L-pieces so that there is at least 1 cm of wax poured around the specimen, to allow for contraction. Pour in melted wax, and embed the object in the plastic skin of cooling wax which forms at the base. As before, take care not to pull down the surface wax.

The watch-glass method lends itself for use with a binocular microscope so that very small specimens can be accurately orientated whilst embedding. Coat the surface of the watch glass with a smear of releasing agent as above, and place under a binocular microscope. Some stands can be arranged so that the watch glass is kept molten on a hot-plate, if preferred. Pour in molten wax and transfer the specimen from the final wax with a flame-polished warmed glass pipette or spatula. Arrange so that the surface to be cut faces downwards in the watchglass.

3.6 Preparation for cutting

Once the block has been removed from the mould, mark the face nearest the tissue with a lightly scored cross using a scalpel or razor. This enables the block to be trimmed (*Figure 3.5*) with reference to the object deep inside, and avoiding cutting through the embedded tissue! Before cutting, soak the surface of the block in ice-water, or other medium listed in Section 4.11.1, if the tissue is at all hard.

Use a single-edged safety razor blade or old microtome knife to trim the block, so that the tissue is central. Leave about 2–3 mm wax around all edges. Pare the wax away, and do not remove too much at once, or the block will crack—usually across the tissue! The sides parallel to the knife edge must themselves be parallel to each other, otherwise good straight ribbons will not form and a disjointed ribbon, or one with a crooked axis, will result. This will cause more problems later when mounting serial sections.

The sides perpendicular to the knife can be trimmed as shown below so that they are either exactly parallel to each other, or else form a trapezium. Where they are parallel it is a good idea to trim one corner to register the correct orientation when mounting the sections later. The height of the block should be trimmed as a truncated pyramid, to provide the maximum support for the cutting face. The short edge of the block should lead, to reduce compression; but if it is cut into a very short edge ribbons may not

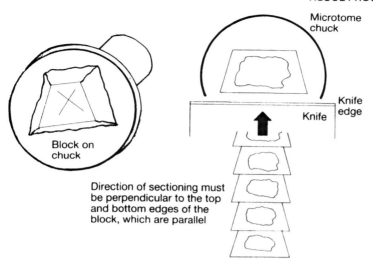

Figure 3.5:   Trimming the wax block. The block should be trimmed in the form of a truncated pyramid (left). The top and bottom sides of the trapezium (right) must be parallel for good ribboning.

occur. The block may either be trimmed before or after mounting on the chuck. Trimming before mounting is best for those microtomes with a vice chuck. Where the chuck is the base-plate and spindle type, mount the block onto the chuck or stub before trimming.

Melt some fresh wax onto a flat spatula or palette knife and press the block onto the plastic wax base. Ensure that the top face to be cut is approximately plane-parallel with the base of the chuck. Buttresses of wax can be built up around the block if it is tall. The block can be slightly cooled under a stream of cold water, but is best left to cool to room temperature over a period of several hours. Rapid overcooling will cause the wax block either to detach or become loose on the chuck, as the coefficients of expansion of wax and metal are different.

3.7 Ribboning

Ribbons will usually form from friction alone as the block is cut, but a low-melting point wax, or mixture of beeswax and embedding wax, may be melted on as a thin layer onto the leading edge of the cutting face. This also assists cutting and manipulating the ribbons when mounting the sections later. As the sections ribbon upon cutting, support the weight of the ribbon without stretching, using forceps to grasp the edge of the leading section. Once the ribbon is the right length, come underneath it with a brush or seeker and gently twist the rear section to one side to peel the trailing edge off the next section. Leave two to three sections on the knife edge to start the next ribbon. It often helps to breathe ('huff') onto each section as it is cut to prevent curling.

3.7.1 Ribboning difficulties

(i)   Sections curl from hard, refractile or brittle tissue—soak or hold the first section section down with a brush as it comes off the knife.
(ii) Reduce static—refer to Section 4.11.2.
(iii) The room atmosphere may be too cold for the wax in use—employ a harder formulation, with a higher melting point, in warm weather and vice versa. Alternatively, the wax may simply be too hard a formulation.
(iv) Wax accretion may have built up on the back of the knife, especially if there was difficulty in getting the first section to cut—clean the back of the knife with xylene and dry thoroughly.
(v)   Embedding may be faulty.
(vi) The sections may be too thick.
(vii) The knife is blunt, tearing minute fibres from the tissue surface.
(viii) The knife tilt may be too great or small—try this adjustment last in this list.

3.7.2 Laying out ribbons

Short ribbons may be placed directly onto a water bath for mounting single sections, as described above. Where serial sections are required, it is best to lay the ribbons onto matt black lining paper contained in a shallow box that has a grooved upper frame to accept a glass lid. Polished (callendered) paper should not be used, as sections will stick to it. When cutting sections from ribbons use a cold curved scalpel blade—they are less likely to stick to the paper when cutting them free.

3.8 Mounting sections onto slides

There are two ways of mounting sections onto slides.

(i)   Directly from the water bath onto the slide and allowing the section to adhere dry over a hot-plate.
(ii) Onto warm fluid over a hot-plate and allowing to dry.

The first method is quicker and simpler: it is most suited where single sections of tissue are required. The second method is better suited to serial sections; it allows the sections to be orientated with respect to one another

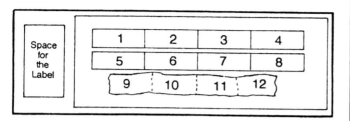

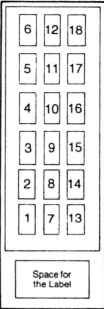

The slide on the left shows paraffin sections. Note the room allowed for the ribbon to stretch. The right-hand slide shows separate sections of LVN, or gelatin cut frozen, mounted individually. Leave space in both cases for the coverslip and label.

Figure 3.6:   Laying out serial sections. It is suggested that serial sections should be laid out, so that with the label to the left they 'read' as text from left to right and top to bottom. Where the slide label is to the bottom of the slide, the sections should be placed in order bottom to top and from left to right.

on the slide, while still removing any wrinkles. The latter method is also better suited to permit stretching of those tissues (e.g. those containing elastin or cysts), which are prone to retaining folds (*Figure 3.6*). The surrounding wax of sections which are collected dry can be cut with a scalpel so that the tissue will stretch unimpeded by the surrounding medium.

3.8.1 The water-bath method

The water bath should be thermostatically controlled, and held at a temperature about 10°C below that of the melting point of the wax. As a rough guide the water should be hot to the touch. If the water is too hot the wax is liable to melt and over-stretch or break up when the section is laid on the water surface, and the morphological arrangement or parts of the section may be lost. If, on the other hand, the water is not sufficiently hot, the section will retain its wrinkles and compressed shape. The same parameters apply to the hot-plate. The water should not be taken straight from the tap, but be boiled and allowed to stand until it reaches the right temperature. In this way, bubbles that could become trapped under the section on the slide will be avoided.

Where tissue is liable to expand at different rates within the section, use a cooler water bath and tease out the wrinkles with forceps and/or seekers. Care should be taken at this stage, as the warm section can very easily stick to the forceps and wrap itself around them as they are lifted free! The problem mainly occurs with cartilage and mucus; blocks with large amounts of these substances should be well-trimmed of free wax before cutting.

Lay the section *matt side up* on the surface of the water bath. The action must be smooth, with the trailing edge of the ribbon touching the water first; the slight dragging that results assists in removing wrinkles. If the layering action is too fast the sections will be overstretched; if too slow the sections will fold up as they are laid down: folds rather than wrinkles are impossible to remove. It is best to cut three or four sections in a ribbon and discard the outer ones once the ribbon has been flattened.

If there is a problem with floating-out, the section can also be laid dry on a microscope slide, which is then flooded with 20% alcohol underneath, and floated onto the water bath where it is picked up in the manner just described. The section to be mounted can then be selected out of the ribbon, and carefully prised apart at the joins using forceps. Move the section to a free edge of the water bath, take a clean grease-free slide and insert the slide into the water at an acute angle of about 60°, a centimeter or so from the section. Do not do this too near the section, or the surface tension of the water as the slide enters will drag the section down into the water. Manoeuvre the slide under the section, and withdraw the slide smoothly in one movement, again at an acute angle, allowing the section to adhere to the slide and be withdrawn.

Shake off the surplus water, and lightly blot with *damp* Postlip blotting paper if required; dry paper will destroy the sections. Moist wax is opaque, while dried sections have transparent wax borders. Label the slide (usually with a diamond marker pen) and dry at 60°C, or just below the melting point of the wax, for 10–30 min on a hot-plate or in the wax oven before dewaxing or storing. Alternatively, the section can be dried off at 37°C overnight (this is good for neural tissue). Other aids to adhesion are: adding gelatin and potassium dichromate separately, from 1% stock solutions, at concentrations of 0.002% to the water-bath; using a slide smeared with a touch of 1% glycerin albumen solution; using slides previously coated with adhesive (Section 7.7).

3.8.2 The hot-plate method

Have the hot-plate pre-warmed so that it is just too hot for the fingertips (if too hot the wax will become filmy and unmanageable). Label the slides and place them on the bars above the hot-plate. It is essential to ensure that the hot-plate is absolutely level. Flood each slide with a small amount of filtered adhesive (e.g. 1% glycerin albumen in distilled water) so that the meniscus of the fluid stands just above the slide.

Cut off sufficient sections to allow for expansion and marking the slide—about a 3 cm length. Pick up the sections with a lightly wetted sable or camel hair brush size 00 or similar. Remove the warmed slide from the hot-plate onto the bench. Place the sections *matt side up* onto the fluid on the warm slide gently and smoothly. Do not drop the sections on, or air bubbles will be trapped underneath.

Transfer the slide to the hot-plate and pipette a little more albumen onto the edge of the slide. Allow the sections to stretch for 10–15 min, but do not allow to dry, or the sections will crinkle. Drying will occur if the surface tension of the albumen or adhesive fluid is broken and it prematurely runs off the slide. Ease out the wrinkles with seekers or forceps. If sections fall on top of one another, or folds occur when laying out cold, they can usually be teased apart, even when wet with albumen, since the ribbon will be stiff.

Once the sections are sufficiently stretched, drain off the excess albumen to a Petri dish, quickly rearrange any sections as required, and let the slides dry over another slightly cooler hot-plate. The sections can be blotted lightly with damp Postlip blotting paper if preferred before drying. Dry blotting paper will tear and lift the sections. For good quality adherence of the sections to the slide transfer the slides to a 40°C oven for 2 days before staining or storage.

3.9 Marking slides

Most slides are plain 76×25 mm slides (3" × 1") 1–1.2 mm (1/23") thick with cut, ground or ground-and-polished edges. The latter type is the best. Slides are available with frosted or plastic-coated surfaces which can be written on in pencil. The most common way is to write on the glass surface with a diamond marker pen. This has the advantage that particles of graphite will not interfere with a sensitive staining (e.g. histochemical) reaction. A diamond marker requires a little practice to use without slipping, but can soon be easily used like a normal pen. An electrical marking pen, the Rotoscriber EDS 20 (Euroserv, UK), is also available.

3.9.1 Locating unstained sections

Sometimes it is possible inadvertently to collect sections onto an unmarked slide, which must be later marked on the correct face. If the slide is held so that the section is viewed in reflected light, then the face with the section uppermost will show a shiny ground and a matt section. If the reverse face is presented to the eye, the entire face, including the section, will appear shiny—indicating that the section is on the obverse face.

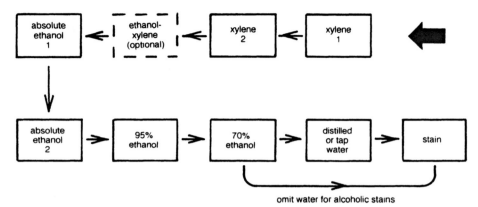

Figure 3.7:   Series of dehydrating and transition media. The 'running down' rehydration series should be kept and used separately from the later dehydration series. Thus this figure is shown separately from *Figure 6.2* to emphasize this fact. Do *not* use one series for both purposes. The ethanol-xylene bath is optional.

3.10 Storing wax blocks

In temperate climates wax blocks will keep indefinitely. Some workers prefer to coat the faced block by dipping briefly into hot paraffin wax before storage. This will keep the tissues from drying out, shrinking and free from predators.

3.11 Rehydrating sections

Paraffin sections are heated after floating out, to cause them first to adhere firmly to the slide, and secondly to melt the wax prior to its removal before staining. Although cold wax will dissolve in xylene, there would otherwise be a risk of residual wax interfering with subsequent staining. The dewaxing and dehydration series is shown in *Figure 3.7*. Care should be taken not to mix the dewaxing xylene and the alcohols on the rehydration series used before staining and the clearing xylene and alcohols of the dehydration series used after staining. This precaution is recommended to prevent wax dissolved in the first series of transition and rehydration media from being deposited in the final mount. The reagents should be changed daily in a busy laboratory, or as soon as the xylene shows signs of supporting wax sediment as a sludge at the bottom of the container. The second xylene and alcohol bath in each case can be moved up and the other reagents replaced with fresh chemicals.

3.12   Gelatin-based embedding media

Tissue which has been fixed and from which frozen sections must be taken (where labile cell products are to be held *in situ*) is best embedded in a protein matrix. The protein solution is solidified, by cross-linking and coagulation, using 25% glutaraldehyde at room temperature. The need to embed specimens in a hot state and then cool them to solidify the block is obviated. The media should be prepared a minimum of 2–3 h in advance, and can be kept for 2–3 weeks in the refrigerator.

Laboratory reagent gelatin	0.75 g
0.1 M phosphate buffer pH 7.3	150 ml
Laboratory reagent powdered egg albumin	57 g
Sucrose	30 g

1. Weigh out the egg albumin into a 500 ml plastic beaker, gradually add 100 ml of buffer. Add the sucrose. Cover the beaker and let the mixture dissolve in the refrigerator overnight. Alternatively, slowly beat the albumin into the buffer until the mixture is homogenous.
2. Rapidly stir 50 ml phosphate buffer in a 200 ml beaker at room temperature, and add the gelatin. Allow to stand for 5 min, then continue to stir while heating to 37°C until dissolved. Allow the gelatin to cool.
3. Mix the albumin and gelatin together, and filter through a double layer of muslin to remove any remaining lumps.

Specimens may be transferred from cold 20% sucrose to the embedding medium. For the best results, infiltrate the tissue overnight at 4°C prior to embedding in fresh medium. Set by adding 0.1 ml 25% glutaraldehyde per 10 ml medium. The mixture will remain sufficiently fluid for 3 min to allow orientation. Use a proprietary non-protein compound instead of a gelatinous medium, for fluorescence work, to avoid non-specific background. Pectin–agar–sucrose is especially useful for fragile specimens: gelatin and agar mixures shrink once frozen, and ice-crystal formation may damage delicate tissues. These phenomena are reduced by the addition of sucrose and pectin, respectively.

Pectin–agar–sucrose

Sucrose	2 g
Agar	2 g
Pectin	2 g
Distilled water	30 ml

Heat to 70–80°C until dissolved. Attach sections to slides with Haupt's gelatin, and dry overnight before staining.

3.13 Other embedding media

Where thin tissues of disparate cell types have to be supported (e.g. retina, monolayer cultures) for thin 3 µm sections, the block can be embedded in a mixture of 2 parts of 20% sucrose in 0.1 M phosphate buffer pH 7.4 to 1 part of proprietary embedding compound. The commercial compounds are a mixture of polyvinyl alcohol and ethylene glycol, and are usually used on their own. For the best results the tissues should be dissected out into fixative, rinsed three times over 30 min in phosphate buffer, and taken through an ascending series of sucrose in phosphate buffer to 20% sucrose overnight at 4°C. Each step should ideally be done on a slow rotator. The tissues should be taken from embedding compound, 1:2, 1:1, and finally 2:1 20% sucrose to embedding compound for 30 min each at 20°C. The material could be orientated in a transparent mould and rapidly snap-frozen in isopentane (2-methyl butane) cooled by liquid nitrogen. The blocks are wrapped in cellophane and aluminium foil and stored at −90°C until needed. Some workers embed tissues in 10%, 20% and finally 25% gelatin after fixing. The block is washed for 3–4 h after 1 day in 10% formalin (to harden the block). Alternatively blocks can be stored until required in the following storage solution.

40% formaldehyde	10 ml
Calcium chloride (anhydrous)	1 g
10% (aq) cadmium chloride	10 ml
Distilled water	80 ml

The cadmium chloride prevents lipid diffusion from the tissue or section.

3.14 Polyethylene glycol (PEG) waxes

PEG formulations, of higher molecular weights than the PEGs used in Tissue-Tek® or other embedding compound for frozen sections, are sometimes employed to avoid using transition media and excessive heat to embed tissues, for example in immunohistochemical studies. PEGs are hygroscopic, waxy solids; these mixtures are also referred to by the trade-name Carbowax®, and the most commonly used mixture is Carbowax 4,000, with a melting point of around 46°C—well below that of paraffin wax. Tissues embedded in PEG often adhere poorly to glass: it may be necessary to use poly-L-lysine- or silane-coated slides, a method for which is given in Gao and Godkin (1991). Klosen *et al.* (1993) report using PEG for immunocytochemistry; these authors embed perfusion-fixed tissues, following dehydration (which appears to conserve antigenicity), in a 30:70% PEG 1000 to PEG 1500 mixture at 46°C, section the material and float out the sections on 0.1 M pH 7.2 Tris-buffered saline.

3.15 Polyester waxes

3.15.1 Ester wax

These waxes comprise esters of glycols using diglycol distearate (DGD) or PEG mixtures. The best known is Steedman's ester wax 1960 mixture (Steedman, 1960), which melts at 48°C. About 4 h are required for tissues to be well impregnated. The waxes are hydrophilic and must not be softened beforehand with water; chill the block in the refrigerator, or stand on the ice-tray with a slip of cellophane in between. For thin sections, it is imperative to cool the block in the refrigerator overnight and to use a cold knife. It is also advisable to cut the sections at a cold ambient temperature—keep breathing on the sections to a minimum. Cut at a temperature between 17 and 27°C with a knife bevel angle of 25°. Prolonged floating of the sections is to be avoided, and the hot-plate method is preferred to the water-bath method of mounting the sections on the slide, as polyester sections will disperse readily in hot water and be lost. Drying must take place at no higher than 37°C.

A suitable embedding protocol is as follows.

1.	70% Cellosolve	8 h
2.	90% Cellosolve	Overnight
3.	Cellosolve I	2.5 h
4.	Cellosolve II	3 h
5.	Cellosolve III	3 h
6.	Cellosolve:Ester wax (50:50) at 37 °C	Overnight
7.	Ester wax I	1 h
8.	Ester wax II	1 h
9.	Ester wax III (vacuum)	1 h
10.	Embed.	

Butan-1-ol (*n*-butyl alcohol) is an alternative transition medium for infiltration, but dewaxing should be carried out with xylene.

3.15.2 Polyester wax

Polyester wax also has a lower melting point (37°C) than conventional paraffin wax, and is alcohol soluble, which makes it suitable for immuno-histochemical studies (Kent, 1991). Polyester waxes must also be sectioned at a much slower rate than paraffin wax, Kent recommends PTFE-coated Ralph knives (Section 4.3.5) used below 22°C. Graham (1982) uses DGD singly, a component of polyester wax, but this is not recommended by Steedman (1960).

3.16 Cellulose embedding

Some confusion can occur with nomenclature. The classical mixture, often used for embedding neural tissues, was celloidin; this has been superseded by LVN. These methods are used for hard and tough tissues, such as uterine wall which is composed of dense connective tissue. Since LVN tissues need only be dehydrated before embedding, and do not need to be heated or passed through a transition medium, it is also the ideal embedding medium for soft and complex tissues which require support and maintenance of different tissue types within the block, such as eyes and neural tissue. Because of its rubbery and homogenous, rather than microcrystalline, structure, LVN sections are slightly more difficult to cut and stain than wax ones, and are cut with a shearing action on a sliding microtome rather than by crack propagation as for wax and resin embedding media.

LVN sections are floated out on a water bath in the same way as decribed for paraffin sections, manipulated on the slide and blotted smooth. They are then stuck to the slide before staining in the following manner. Dip the slide into 0.5% LVN in a 50:50% ether to ethanol mixture for a few seconds, drain, and wipe the back of the slide. The section can also be stuck to the slide by pouring ether fumes over the section, but the former method is easier to use in a fume hood. Immerse the slide in chloroform for 5–10 min, to harden the celloidin, and dehydrate via the alcohols to 70%. Take the section directly to stain, if this contains alcohol, or else wash the section in water before transferring to aqueous stains. Other workers prefer to stain the free-floating sections (Section 6.5) before mounting them on the slide. If xylene is used as the transition medium prior to mounting, it will be noticed that the xylene does not dissolve the LVN, as it does wax, but renders it transparent.

Nitrocellulose is supplied like wool dampened with butanol, since it is explosive when dry. The solutions should be made up a week in advance, since they (celloidin in particular) take a long time to dissolve. Once dissolved, the stock should be diluted with an equal quantity of ether. Store the solutions in jars with ground glass stoppers to prevent solvent evaporation, and contamination with water.

Thin solution	5% LVN or 2% celloidin in ethanol/ether
Medium solution	10% LVN or 4% celloidin in ethanol/ether
Thick solution	20% LVN or 8% celloidin in ethanol/ether

Tissues should ideally be no more than 10 mm thick, and infiltrated under vacuum (–400 to –500 mmHg). The tissue will appear to be 'boiling' at this stage. The vacuum should be applied daily for 10–30 min, and the block infiltrated until the celloidin is rubbery, and just resists thumbnail pressure. The tissues can be left in the embedding medium almost indefinitely, provided that it is not allowed to evaporate. The specimen can be orientated at this stage on a partially hardened layer of medium, and fresh medium poured in. Once rubbery, the block can be hardened by exchange of the ethanol–ether in chloroform vapour for up to 24 h. The chloroform vapour step can be omitted, and the blocks hardened solely by evaporation, or rapid hardening may be affected in a few hours using a chloroform solution. Both chloroform techniques result in harder, tougher blocks than by evaporation alone. Most workers store the blocks in 70% ethanol until required for sectioning; Gray (1954) recommends storage in chloroform. Lillie and Fullmer (1976) suggest that the block is transferred via a stepwise (3:1, 1:1, 1:3) chloroform-to-cedarwood oil mixture, and kept in 100% cedarwood oil for at least 24 h prior to cutting. If double embedding (e.g. Peterfi's method) is envisaged, the infiltration should proceed as given below.

3.16.1 Double embedding

The use of heat is in direct opposition to the aims of celloidin embedding, and these methods have largely been superseded by embedding in resins which are polymerized *in situ* rather than by evaporation of the solvent. Sections embedded in cellulose media may tend to curl as they are cut (Section 4.8.4) and can be floated onto an alcohol bath. It is necessary to use albumen, or another of the adhesives in Section 7.7, for the best results. Some workers prefer to include a 95% alcohol step in the dehydration series. Toluene, rather than chloroform, is used to harden the tissues (to prevent brittleness). The wax should not be heated to higher than 60°C, otherwise the tissue blocks will be difficult to section.

Peterfi's method

1.	Transfer the tissue to 70% ethanol	Overnight
2.	90% ethanol	4 h
3.	Absolute ethanol	4 h
4.	1% celloidin in methyl salicilate I	24 h
5.	1% celloidin in methyl salicilate II	24 h
6.	1% celloidin in methyl salicilate III	24 h
7.	Toluene I	8 h
8.	Toluene II	8 h
9.	Toluene III	8 h
10.	Paraffin wax I	2 h
11.	Paraffin wax II	3 h
12.	Paraffin wax III	3 h

Disadvantages of nitrocellulose embedding
(i)   It is difficult to cut sections thinner than 10 µm.
(ii)   Ribboning is impossible, so collecting serial sections is tedious.
(iii)   Processing is relatively slow, making it difficult for routine work.
(iv)   Blocks and sections must be stored in 70% alcohol in the dark; this is hazardous and consumes space.
(v)   Ether is used as a solvent; it is extremely flammable—extinguish all naked lights before use.

These disavantages have meant that to a large extent the use of nitrocellulose has been superseded by resins. Another possibility is to embed tissues with polystyrene in toluene (Frangioni and Borgioli, 1979). The authors claim that the advantages of celloidin embedding for heterogenous tissues, the ease of preparation and staining of paraffin sections and the thinness of resin sections, are all retained in one method. However, it has not been widely accepted.

3.17 Orientation of small objects whilst embedding

It is sometimes necesssary to control precisely the manner in which tissues are embedded. This may be either because the specimens are very small, and their position must be known precisely for effective sectioning, or because sectioning involves the reduction of a three-dimensional specimen to a series of two dimensions, and the plane of reduction must be known.

The simplest way to hold a flat piece of tissue (e.g. retina) in place for sectioning is to embed it between slices of formalin-fixed, alcohol-hardened liver, which is then bound around the tissue with thread and taken through as a sandwich until the last change of wax. The thread is cut just before embedding the whole as a wax block. For most purposes it is sufficient to keep the wax molten using a heated stage or hot-plate, and use a dissecting microscope to manipulate the specimen into place with warm tools. For best results a thin layer of fresh wax is allowed to just solidify, and the object cast within fresh wax poured on top of this layer. If a hot-plate is not available, a specially designed heating filament has been described by Hilger and Medan (1987).

Most other methods for precise orientation involve embedding specimens in a porous mesh of agar (Arnolds, 1978), or albumen cold-set with glutaraldehyde (Section 3.12). Janisch (1974) reports a method which includes a marker strip of black paper to locate the specimen which may be invisible to the naked eye. Where embedding in agar will dilute the specimen (e.g. cell suspensions) it is possible to preform a frothy layer of agar on a slide, and cast the suspension in a drop of molten agar within a suitable bubble (Hernández-Mariné, 1992). Most transition media used for paraffin will destroy the agar block, and so either dioxan or amyl acetate must be used (Buzzell, 1975).

Orientation methods for water-miscible acrylic resin embedding may also employ agar (Ridgway and Chestnut, 1984). Pieces of unexposed photographic film are developed, fixed and washed; circles are then punched out with a hole punch. Two parallel slits are cut at one edge, and the handling tab (which also serves as a reference point) is bent upwards. The specimen is orientated and set into a drop of 2% solution of agar pipetted on the circle. The drop is cooled to cause gelling, and then positioned horizontally into a size 00 gelatin capsule part-filled with resin. The capsule is topped up and polymerized. Before sectioning, the gelatin is dissolved or cut away, and the film disc removed to reveal the orientated specimen.

Where specimens are to be embedded in water-immiscible epoxy resins, or are flat or elongated, either a flat electron microscope mould or the method of Prentø (1985) is suitable. With the latter technique a size 00 electron microscope polythene capsule is capped, laid on its side and the top part of the body cut away. The 'drum' so formed is three-quarters filled with resin and prepolymerized for 16 h at 40°C. The specimen is then orientated in a drop of resin (prewarmed at 40°C to thin it), the capsule topped up and polymerization completed for 2 days at 60°C.

Another method (Sene, 1991), suitable for reconstructing epoxy resin serial sections, can be adapted for orientating the specimen prior to sectioning. Essentially, the specimen is embedded in a drop of medium over a groove in a silicone mould. Once set, the block is inverted and the protruding tab covered with stained resin. The combined block is re-embedded and sectioned transversely to the tab, which serves to locate the specimen.

When tissues are stained for immunohistochemistry, several serial sections are often mounted on multi-spot slides (C. A. Hendley, Essex), so that fewer slides are processed at any one time, saving reagents and permitting comparisons between sections. Miller and Groothuis (1991) describe a method whereby thin paraffin-embedded strips of different tissues may be incorporated into a 'sausage' block; 3–5 mm slices of this sausage are then re-embedded and sections cut and mounted in the normal way. This method works best with homogeneous tissues of similar density.

3.18 Resin embedding media

The ubiquitous paraffin wax has four important disadvantages which necessitate the use of resins. It is rarely possible to cut good quality paraffin sections below 2 μm, and paraffin does not offer adequate support for sectioning hard tissues, which will tear out of soft media. Although it is possible to carry out combined light/electron microscope studies on paraffin sections (Johannessen, 1977), it is simpler to use a resin which will permit semi-thin and ultra-thin sections to be cut from the same block. Thirdly, tissues embedded in paraffin wax shrink by a greater proportion than those embedded in resin. Shrinkage of various pure resins has been reported as about 3% for epoxy and 15% for acrylic resins—the shrinkage of the infiltrated tissue is less than this because the tissue provides further resistance to shrinkage. These are values recorded after polymerization. Nevertheless it is possible to use resins which cure at a low temperature to reduce further the shrinkage that may occur at this step in tissue processing. Fourthly, some hydrophilic resins allow the direct use of aqueous stains without the need for employing transition media.

It is worth noting that while tissue embedded in paraffin wax can be reclaimed if poorly processed, or can be re-embedded in a different orientation, this is almost impossible to do with blocks impregnated in resin (see Hayat, 1989 for two methods). In addition, for most acrylic resins, the polymerization reaction is strongly exothermic, which is a disadvantage for some labile tissue components (e.g. antigens). For this reason, resins which can be cured at low temperature have been developed (Section 3.18.3); it is however possible to demonstrate some antigens in sections of Araldite or glycol methacrylate (GMA) resin which has been cured above 0°C. The reader is referred to Britten *et al.* (1993) for a comparative study.

When using a new batch of resin, a control block of tissue should be processed (as is done for new batches of dyes and staining solutions) to ensure that no variation of the formulation or protocol is required. The shelf-life of acrylic monomers is often short: accelerators should not be kept for longer than 6 months. Most embedding problems can be traced to old constituents, particularly those which have become hydrated.

Not only should minimal stocks be kept, it is also unwise to mix more resin than is needed for immediate use, although some workers, particularly with viscous resins, will mix a large quantity and store it at −20°C for re-use. Not only does the resin become more viscous each time it is used, but if used cold will condense water onto the surface of the block. Some resins are extremely sensitive to excess water either from condensation on removal from the refrigerator, humid atmosphere, old hydrated monomer or residual water in the processed tissue. Where gelatin capsules are used to exclude oxygen during embedding, these should be heated gently in an incubator to dry them thoroughly before use.

There is a wide range of synthetic resins available to the histologist. This text will deal only with selected representative examples intended for light microscopy. The different types of resins can be classed as follows.

(i)	Epoxy	(Araldite, Epon, Spurr's)
(ii)	Acrylic	(GMA, LR resins, Unicryl, JB-4, Lowicryls)
(iii)	Polyester	(Vestopal W)

Some of these resins, most of which have been formulated for transmission electron microscopy, are designed to be used at low temperatures for preservation of antigens and other labile cellular structures.

The components, as well as dust from the partly cured resins, present considerable hazards. The reader is strongly advised to refer to Causton *et al.* (1981) and Tobler and Freiburghaus (1990) for safety details concerning the use of synthetic resins and storage of the monomeric constituents. In a later article, Causton (1988) gives a useful summary table detailing the safe handling of resin components. Gloves should be worn at all times when handling resins. If two pairs are worn, one on top of the other, not only is further protection given, but the outer glove can be changed easily when it becomes contaminated. Wear nitrile gloves for epoxy resins and vinyl gloves for acrylics. Remove skin contamination using soap and *cold* water. Do not use solvents. An apparatus for minimizing exposure to the dehydration and infiltration reagents used in resin embedding has been devised by Redmond and Bob (1984).

3.18.1 Epoxy resins

These mixtures are hardened using cross-linking anhydrides accelerated by amines, usually at 60°C. Commonly used for electron microscopy, they are the hardest of the resin formulae employed in microscopy. The consistency of the block may be modified by flexibilizers and plasticizers, which reduce hardness and brittleness and increase tensile strength. Flexibilizers are incorporated into the cross-linked structure of the block, while plasticizers are not. Araldite and Epon resins have been formulated principally for electron microscopy and do not adapt well to larger blocks for light microscopy. The components may be measured gravimetrically, or preferably by volume. The accelerator should be measured very accurately, to 0.1 g or 0.1 ml. Resin sections are prone to lifting from the slide, with consequent wrinkles and folds, although this can be reduced by drying under a vacuum for 24–48 h. Furthermore, semi-thin sections of epoxy resins, being water immiscible, do not accept a large repertoire of stains, the most commonly used oversight stains are toluidine blue and Azure II-methylene blue (Section 6.5.3). Some workers suggest that wrinkles and folds occur during staining rather than while the sections are drying. To obviate this effect, Sommer *et al.* (1979) dissolve the dye in 50% glycerol, and stain for 12–24 h in a covered dish.

Araldite resin

4,4′Isopropylidenediphenol (Araldite M, CY212) (diglycidyl ether of bisphenol A)	Resin	40 parts
Dodecenyl succinic anhydride (DDSA, HY964/964B)	Hardener	40 parts
Benzyl dimethylamine (BDMA, DY062)	Accelerator	2.3 parts

The plasticizer dibutyl phthalate (DBP) comprises 19% by weight of Araldite CY212, but Araldite MY753 and Araldite 502 contain only

17% DBP. If these are substituted in the above protocol, 1 part of DBP should be added. A softer block is best adjusted by trial and error using the flexibilizer DER 736, adding 1 ml to start with. The original accelerator used was 2,4,6-tris(dimethylaminomethyl)phenol (DMP-30, DY064/964C). Since DMP-30 has a short shelf-life, is more viscous than BDMA, is inactivated by exposure to water vapour, and is the usual culprit of inadequate embedding, it is now not used so much, BDMA being preferable. Both accelerators give off toxic fumes when heated. Replacing each ml of the DDSA with 0.5 ml methyl Nadic anhydride will give harder blocks than the formulation above. Epon resins are similar to Araldite and are based on triglycidyl ether of glycerol, rather than diglycidyl ether of bisphenol A, as the resin monomer. Suitable protocols for using Epon and Epon/Araldite mixtures, and an excellent review of the use of epoxy resins may be found in Glauert (1991).

Spurr's resin is the best epoxy resin suited to light microscopy being of low viscosity (60 cP at 25°C), but it has the disadvantage of being extremely toxic, and volatile, and may cause contact sensitivity. The resin ERL 4206 is a known carcinogen.

Spurr's resin

Vinyl cyclohexane dioxide (ERL 4206)	Resin	10 parts
Polypropylene glycol diglycidyl ether (DER 736)	Flexibilizer	6 parts
Nonenyl succinic anhydride (NSA)	Hardener	26 parts
Dimethylaminoethanol (S-1)	Accelerator	0.4 parts

Use 4 parts of DER 736 for a harder block, and 8 parts for a softer block.

The rate at which the block is cured will also affect its final properties, according to the number of cross-links that are formed. Rapid curing at a high temperature will form a hard, brittle block that is highly impervious to aqueous stains. Conversely, slower polymerization at a lower temperature will produce a softer block that may need more care in sectioning, but will be more amenable to staining. For further details on the molecular structure of epoxy resins, and the way in which cross-linking affects the properties of resins, the reader is referred to Causton (1980).

Epoxy resin mixtures which contain accelerators are very hygroscopic, and so the alcohol, transition agent and resin monomer must be absolutely dry. Propylene oxide is used as the transition medium—in general a softer block than that required for electron microscopy will be needed, and the reader is referred to Janes (1979) for further details. Providing that the sections are well dried for about 30–60 min on a hot-plate at 60°C, there should be few problems with wrinkles or folds occurring. If problems persist, it may help to try the vacuum drying method reported by Crowley and Leichtling (1989) or the remedies suggested by Horobin (1989).

General epoxy resin embedding protocol
1. Fix tissues as required; wash with running water or two washes of buffer for 30 min.

2. Dehydrate tissues through an ascending aqueous ethanol or acetone series, starting with 30%, then 50%, 70%, 90%, 100% and two (dry) 100% washes, all for 10–15 min at the temperature used for fixation.
3. Pre-warm and pre-mix the resin, hardener and flexibilizer (if used) at 60°C. Allow several minutes for the bubbles to disperse. Some workers store these components mixed. Mixing the components well before the addition of accelerator gives a more transparent block.
4. Measure out the resin by weight, or by volume using a warm glass cylinder, into a warm disposable beaker and swirl to mix very well. Drain the cylinder at 60°C and add the accelerator.
5. Infiltrate the tissue with resin-acetone or (if ethanol has been used) resin-propylene oxide in an increasing ratio. Use the ratios 1:3, 1:1, 3:1 and two changes of fresh resin before embedding. Epoxy resins infiltrate slowly, so each step must be at least an hour, preferably using a shaker or rotator. Most workers leave the specimens in the 1:1, or preferably 1:3, mixture overnight at 4°C.
6. Cure Araldite at 60°C for 1–3 days (some workers prefer the first day at 40°C); Epon mixtures at 60°C for 2–3 days and Spurr's resin at 70°C for 8 h or 60°C for 20 h.

It is safest, for both knife and microtomist, to cast blocks in disposable plastic moulds; take care with cutting these away with scalpels or single-edged razor blades. If a glass container is used to cast the block, either smash it wrapped in a thick cloth or submerged in a bucket of water, and wear eye protection.

A technique for embedding large specimens for light microscopy into epoxy resin has been published by Anker *et al.* (1974), who embed at 4°C under periodic vacuum. Epoxy resin blocks may be sectioned to provide ribbons for light microscopy (Richards, 1980) by double embedding with a secondary epoxy resin and very hard PEG 6000. The tissues are cut dry and mounted onto the slides with acetone, where the original sections flatten and the secondary mixture dissolves.

3.18.2 Acrylic resins

GMA (2-hydroxyethylmethacrylate, HEMA), is the best known and most commonly used resin mixture (Litwin, 1985; Murray, 1988). GMA (50 centipoise at 25°C) is less viscous than either methyl methacrylate (MMA) or epoxy resin, so that larger blocks can be cast in a shorter time, and less non-specific background results when acrylics are used for immunological studies. Moreover, the GMA monomer is water-miscible and the polymer water-permeable, and is less likely than MMA resin to cause disruption of tissues due to gas bubble formation. Dehydration and transition using solvents can therefore be dispensed with, and infiltration commenced with 70% aqueous GMA (see below). Three earlier, important reviews on the use of acrylic resins in animal and plant histology have been published by

Bennett *et al.* (1976) and Feder and O'Brien (1968), Ameele (1976), respectively.

MMA.   MMA is miscible with both acetone and ethanol, and is particularly suitable (on its own or with GMA) for embedding both mineralized and decalcified bone and other hard tissues. The sections must be attached to the slide with adhesive, and etched for staining. Polymerization is extremely exothermic, and will proceed spontaneously in light; therefore, methacrylate resins are sold with 0.1% methoxy ethyl hydroquinone inhibitors, which do not usually affect the quality of the final block. Benzoyl peroxide (BPO) is used to initiate polymerization; it should be used within 6 months of manufacture. Dry BPO is explosive, and so is commonly supplied dampened or as a 50% paste in dibutyl phthalate.

MMA embedding medium

MMA	Resin monomer	10 ml
BPO	Initiator	0.05 g
Nonylphenol polyglycol etheracetate	Plasticizer	1 ml
N'N-dimethylaniline (DMA)	Activator	50 µl

MMA embedding protocol
1. Fixation of specimens up to 5 mm thick should be for 12–24 h.
2. The specimens can be dehydrated to 95% ethanol, transferred to an equal mixture of 95% ethanol and resin without the activator (all steps for 12 h minimum).
3. Infiltrate with the resin (excluding activator) under vacuum (8–10 kPa), with three changes of fresh resin for 12–24 h, depending upon the size of the block. If over 1 cm^3, double these recommended times. Embed in fresh resin, including activator.
4. Polymerize dry in a water bath at 37°C for 24–72 h. In cool climates, polymerization may be initiated by heating at 47°C for 30 min.

Unicryl® is a water-miscible acrylic resin available from British Biocell International as a single solution, and is suitable for light and electron microscopy. It comprises a mixture of methacrylate monomers and styrene (Scala *et al.*, 1992) of low viscosity, which can be cured by heat at 55°C for 1–2 days or UV radiation.

GMA.   Conventional acrylics are polymerized by a radical addition chain reaction, which breaks the acrylic double bond. Radical scavengers such as oxygen and acetone should be avoided, since they will stop the polymerization. BPO is used as the source of radicals, and with the addition of tertiary aromatic amines (dimethyl aniline) will initiate polymerization at 0°C. Slower, rather than faster, polymerization will give a tough block that is easy to section, and (due to fewer cross-links) one which will be better penetrated by aqueous reagents.

GMA embedding protocol (Gerrits et al., *1987)*

GMA, HEMA	Resin	90 ml

2-Butoxyethanol, ethylene glycol monobutyl ether	Plasticizer	10 ml
BPO (moistened with 20% water)		0.5 g

Accelerating medium

PEG 200 or 400 (plasticizer)	Carrier for accelerator	15 ml
DMA	Accelerator	1 ml

GMA embedding routine

1. Fix specimens of 10×5 mm maximum size in neutralized or pH 7.4 0.1 M phosphate-buffered formalin prepared from paraformaldehyde (without methanol additive) for 6–12 h.
2. Dehydrate the tissue in 70% ethanol for 1 h, then in two changes of 95% ethanol for 2 h and absolute ethanol for 1 h.
3. Pre-infiltrate the tissue with an equal mixture of absolute ethanol and embedding medium for 2 h. Infiltrate the tissue overnight in fresh embedding medium.
4. Infiltrate with resin, two changes for 1 day each; the second change under light vacuum. Cover with a thin layer of paraffin oil to exclude oxygen.
5. Embed the tissues using a Teflon embedding mould in a 30:1 mixture of embedding to accelerating medium which has previously been mixed for 1 min at room temperature. Initiated solutions can be made up and kept for up to eight weeks, if stored at 4°C. This helps to reduce incomplete infiltration and polymerization.
6. Polymerize under UV for 2 days, or at 60°C for 3 days, or 70°C for 12 h. Glue the block to the microtome chuck with Araldite for 5 min.

The components can be mixed by hand using an orange stick, but there is less risk of introducing air bubbles with a magnet stirrer. The mixed resin can be stored for 1 month at room temperature. If stored in a refrigerator, the BPO will separate out and must be stirred in again before use.

Dehydration is only required up to 95% alcohol, as the final resin contains 6–8% water. For uniform penetration use an intermediate mixture of equal parts of resin with 95% ethanol as an intermediate step between the dehydration and infiltration. Polymerization will take up to 2 h at room temperature, with large, dense or fatty specimens requiring longer, often at 4–10°C overnight. Lung, botanical and similar vacuolated specimens should be infiltrated under slight vacuum. Polymerization will start to occur within 30 min, and is faster for larger volumes; therefore, prepare the smallest volume of resin that is needed for the job. Because GMA monomers are hygroscopic, polymerization in a humid atmosphere will create soft blocks which are difficult to section. In this case, the amount of embedding resin should be reduced.

Embedding in pre-polymerized resin is used by some workers to reduce the formation of swelling artifacts. The monomers are completely dissolved at 40°C, and heated to 98°C at the rate of $7°C \, min^{-1}$ while stirring. At this temperature the resin is rapidly cooled in a dry ice–ethanol bath to about 2°C, after which it may be frozen and stored indefinitely. For large blocks, slightly different, softer, GMA formulae have been published by Sims (1974) and Murgatroyd (1976) which will permit sectioning on rotary as well as sledge microtomes. GMA resin can also be purchased in kit form (e.g. JB-4), most of which contain no methacrylic acid, a contaminant responsible for heavy background staining in the resin. A processing schedule for JB-4 resin is given in Stevens and Germain (1990).

Sectioning.   Pick the section off the knife (a pointed 'tongue' on one edge of the block as illustrated by Sims (1974) may help), and transfer it to a water bath, or a drop of water on a slide. The section should flatten immediately. If there is any tendency for the section to wrinkle or fold, dunk it into absolute alcohol and then into a water bath. The section can then be floated onto a clean slide, wiped around, and heat-dried onto the slide at 60°C for 30 min. Double embedding in a resin/PEG mixture according to Richards (1980) will allow ribbons of serial sections to be cut.

Where differentiation of GMA-embedded tissue is required, particularly after the use of basic dyes at neutral pH, the sections can be differentiated in the following mixture.

GMA monomer	30 ml
Butan-1-ol (*n*-butanol)	30 ml
Acetone	30 ml
Distilled water	1 ml

1. Dry the sections on a hot-plate in the normal way.
2. Differentiate at room temperature as required.   5–10 min
3. Rinse in butan-1-ol.
4. Transfer through xylene and mount in DPX.

3.18.3 Lowicryl and London resins

Lowicryl resins were principally developed as low-viscosity resins for low-temperature embedding immunocytochemistry (Acetarin *et al.*, 1986; Altman *et al.*, 1984; Ashford, 1986; Newman, 1987) by the Chemie Werke Lowi GmbH. They are usually polymerized by UV light but can also be heat-cured. Lowicryl HM20 and HM23 are hydrophobic embedding media; K4M and K11M polar, hydrophilic media. In this case, the polarity of K4M and K11M refers to the ability of the resins to preserve, in embedded tissue, the structural polarity that naturally occurs in the protein component of tissues. K4M is the principal Lowicryl resin used for light microscopy and will polymerize with 5% residual water. However, it is less suited to embedding pigmented material, especially plants, which absorb strongly at 360 nm, the wavelength of UV light used to cure the resin.

The depth of penetration of UV radiation into tissues is limited, about 0.07 mm. Therefore, specimens must be very small (about 1 mm^3) and polymerization should ideally be unilateral. Suitable apparatus for polymerization has been constructed by Rostgaard and Buchmann (1974) for UV, and Nuttall (1986) for white light. Alternatively, the gelatin capsules can be supported in a plastic support on a glass plate above the light source. A typical UV radiation protocol is as follows: 100 W tungsten-halogen lamp at 20 cm or 2×8 W UV lamps at 15 cm for 24 h at $-30°C$, then 2–3 days at room temperature. Oxygen will inhibit polymerization, particularly if heat-cured using benzoyl ethyl ether; therefore, use a nitrogen atmosphere, and/or stir the components gently. These resins are primarily used for electron microscopy.

LR White and LR Gold are produced by the London Resin Company— hence the name—and are aromatic polyhydroxy dimethacrylate compounds which are not only hydrophilic and of low viscosity (8 cP), but are also stable in an electron beam. They are therefore useful for joint light/electron microscopy studies (Newman and Hobot, 1987). LR White is less suited for low temperature embedding for immunohistochemistry because the exothermic chemical accelerator may cause localized extreme temperature rises. LR White comes in three grades (hard, medium, soft) to match the hardness of the tissue to be embedded, and the acrylic monomers can be stored at $4°C$ for up to a year. The resin is compatible with up to 12% residual water in tissues. Sections should be collected as soon as possible due to the hydrophilic nature of the resin.

Protocol for LR White
1. Fix as given above.
2. Dehydrate through an increasing aqueous ethanol sequence, starting with 30% ethanol, to absolute ethanol. Do not use acetone, which will interfere with curing.
3. Infiltrate 1 mm^3 blocks with three changes of resin for 1 h each (at room temperature or $4°C$), or leave at $4°C$ overnight.
4. Polymerize at $50 \pm 2°C$ for 48 h, excluding oxygen using gelatin capsules, paraffin oil, or a nitrogen-rich atmosphere. The block quality is more susceptible than epoxy resin to variations in polymerization. If cold curing, add 15 μl of accelerator to 10 ml of resin and leave for 15 min in a cold water bath to dissipate the heat produced. Exclude as much oxygen as possible during polymerization, and use gelatin capsules, since air will permeate polyethylene moulds.
5. Float the sections on 70% alcohol, or 40% acetone with 1% benzyl alcohol, on a hot-plate at $60°C$, and dry for 1 h.
7. After staining, since LR White is softened by alcohol, blot the sections, dry on a hot-plate at $60°C$, and either mount from xylene into a resinous mountant or directly into LR White with 1 drop accelerator per ml, as a mountant. (This mountant will gel within 2 min).

If hard tissue is defatted with chloroform after dehydration, the tissue should be returned to absolute ethanol to remove the chloroform before resin infiltration. Despite the narrow range of polymerization temperature quoted by the manufacturers, there has been a report (Hillmer *et al.*, 1991) on the use of microwaves to cure LR White blocks. Since the polymerization reaction is strongly exothermic, and may damage tissues, the concentration of added initiator is critical to allow adequate polymerization and yet prevent strongly exothermic reactions. Osmium tetroxide should be avoided in critical studies, as it may absorb heat causing focal 'hot-spots' resulting in loss of antigenicity. Similarly, yellow pigments may selectively absorb UV radiation causing unevenly polymerized blocks. Protocols for Lowicryl resins and LR Gold are given in Stevens and Germain (1990) and Smith and Croft (1991).

3.19 Resin removal

Unless the resin is hydrophilic or, like GMA, of a similar structure to wax, then aqueous stains will not penetrate easily. While GMA monomer is miscible with water, its polymer is insoluble, and so cannot be removed from sections. Furthermore, basic (cationic) dyes are taken up strongly by GMA at neutral pH, reducing contrast between tissue and resin. Methacrylate resins, however, can easily be dissolved from sections by immersion in acetone for a few seconds. Staining times often have to be increased or modified, or the resin has to be extracted from the section using sodium ethoxide. This solution will go brown after a few days, but it has a long shelf-life.

Sodium hydroxide   2 g
Absolute ethanol   100 ml

1. Dissolve the sodium hydroxide in the ethanol, and stand overnight.
2. Immerse sections in the solution at 20–26°C for 1 h.
3. Follow with a vigorous water wash for 15 min.
4. Stain.
5. Air-dry and mount directly in resin medium.

3.20 Methods for hard tissues

Most tissues require hardening by fixation before they can be sectioned adequately. There are, however, three major categories of tissues which need softening, following stabilization of their cellular component by fixation, before sectioning: the calcified tissues found in animal histology, the lignified woody tissues encountered in botany and the chitinous exoskeleton of insects. Other materials (hair, diatom frustules) may be examined without such treatment.

3.20.1 Decalcification

For our purposes, the mineral calcium of bones can be considered as hydroxyapatite; calcium ions are removed through the action of hydrogen ions (the equation is considered in Kiernan, 1990). The decalcifying fluids (*Table 3.1*) must therefore be changed frequently to remove these ions, and drive the equation to completion. The most common acids used are hydrochloric, nitric and formic acids. Although mineral acids will fix the tissues, prior fixation is mandatory for good results, and prevents the swelling and displacement of the undenatured collagen and other protein components of the bone. Excess skin should be removed, and large specimens sawn into slices. The resulting debris should be washed away under a gentle stream of distilled water to prevent its being embedded into the tissue.

Table 3.1:   Decalcifying agents

1 M nitric acid	
Concentrated nitric acid (sp. gr. 1.42; 70% w/w)	63 ml
Distilled water to	1000 ml
1 M hydrochloric acid [a]	
Concentrated hydrochloric acid (sp. gr. 1.18; 36% w/w)	86 ml
Distilled water to	1000 ml
4 M formic acid	
Concentrated formic acid (sp. gr. 1.21; 90% w/w)	170 ml
Distilled water to	1000 ml
Buffered formic acid [b]	
Concentrated formic acid (sp. gr. 1.21; 90% w/w)	271 ml
Sodium hydroxide	19.8 g
Distilled water to	1000 ml
de Castro's fluid [c]	
Absolute ethanol	300 ml
Chloral hydrate	50 g
Distilled water to	1000 ml
Concentrated nitric acid (sp. gr. 1.42; 70% w/w)	30 ml
Pereyeni's fluid [d]	
10% aqueous nitric acid	40 ml
Absolute ethanol	30 ml
0.5% aqueous chromium trioxide	30 ml
EDTA [e]	
EDTA (pH to 7.4 with approximately 280 ml 1 M NaOH)	100 g
Distilled water to	1000 ml

[a] Alter these concentrations to 10% for old, and 1–2% for developing, bone.
[b] This mixture (pH 2.0) is favoured by Brain (1966) when there is no urgency for results. It will keep indefinitely once made up.
[c] These reagents *must* be mixed in the order stated. Concentrated nitric acid reacts explosively with ethanol. The pH is about 1.0. de Castro's fluid may be used as a combined fixing and decalcifying mixture.
[d] Prepare this mixture just before use.
[e] EDTA is a chelating agent which should be made up freshly before use. It has the advantage that carbon dioxide is not liberated from the tissues, with the consequent risk of distortion.

Strong mineral acids act very rapidly, in 1–2 days, while the organic chelating agent ethylenediaminetetra-acetic acid disodium salt (EDTA) will take several weeks. It is important to determine the end-point of decalcification so that tissues are not destroyed, and the ability of basiphilic chromatin to stain is not depleted. Secondary fixation (Section 2.8) can ameliorate these effects to some extent, and if chosen the tissue should be rinsed and blotted after decalcification before proceeding with secondary fixation. The most commonly used strong mineral acid is nitric acid, which causes less swelling than hydrochloric acid. The acid should not be added in its concentrated form to ethanol, with which it will react explosively. When using a mild decalcifier, formic acid is often used for all specimens except dense cortical bone.

With any of these decalcifying solutions the following procedure is used (Brain, 1966).

1. Reduce the thickness of the specimen so that this does not exceed 3 mm.
2. Place it on a bed of non-adherent lint in a 250 ml flask.
3. Cover the specimen with 250 ml of fluid and cover the top with foil, parafilm, or a cotton wool plug. The temperature should be kept to about 18–25°C, unless using EDTA when temperatures up to 60°C can be used. If elevated temperatures are used with acids, there is a high risk that the tissues will be macerated.
4. Change strong mineral acids two or three times a day, and other fluids daily. Test the system daily for end-point determination.

Saturated aqueous picric acid is useful for the decalcification of developing bones, but requires frequent changing. Lactic acid can be used as a 2 M solution, and like formic acid will take up to 3 weeks to decalcify tissue, but both give excellent tissue preservation and nuclear staining. Acetic, oxalic, phosphoric, sulphuric and tartaric acids are to be avoided; they either act very slowly and swell tissues unacceptably, or else impair nuclear staining. Citric acid is not usually used alone because it is too slow; however, Foschini and Muzzi (1993) describe its use as a decalcifying fluid to preserve certain antigens. Alternatively, for immunohistochemical studies, frozen sections of undecalcified bone may be used (Hill and Elde, 1990). Decalcifying mixtures which contain large amounts of alcohol to counteract any swelling due to the acid, tend to cause distortion and will, in any case, suppress decalcification by retarding the formation and solution of mineral ions.

3.20.2 Determination of end-point

It is important to determine the end-point accurately and reliably, since the rate of decalcification will differ from one specimen to another depending upon the amount of mineralized tissue and its accessibility within the connective tissue matrix of the bone. If decalcification is prolonged, tissue morphology and nuclear staining will suffer as swelling, maceration and acidophilic bias ensue. If the process is not completed, then microtomy will be difficult, and the knife may well be ruined.

Calcium oxalate test

Concentrated ammonia solution	10 ml
Saturated aqueous (about 6%) ammonium oxalate	5 ml

1. Commence the test 24 h after the first immersion. Mix the decalcifying fluid, and take off a 5 ml aliquot.
2. Add 1 ml ammonia solution and mix well. If a precipitate is seen there is no need to proceed. Change the decalcifying fluid and test again after 24 h, if no precipitate is seen.
3. Add 0.1 ml ammonium oxalate, and if there is no precipitate, leave the solution for 20 min. Add two further aliquots of ammonium oxalate at 20 min intervals until a precipitate is seen, or the solution remains clear—indicating that decalcification is complete.

Calcium oxalate will not precipitate from acid mixtures which are greater than 0.7 M or less than pH 4.5. Therefore, higher concentrations must be diluted before testing.

Once the tissues are decalcified, they must be washed thoroughly to prevent contamination of the dehydrating agents, particularly if an automatic carousel containing several different types of tissue is used. Specimens up to 3 mm thick should be washed for 2–4 h, while those up to 9 mm thick require 12–15 h, or until the pH is that of the wash water alone. It is sufficient to wash them in 500 ml of distilled water which is changed hourly or so. Automatic continuous washing equipment should not be used where damage to the soft decalcified tissue may result.

3.20.3 Sectioning

A heavy microtome and tungsten carbide knife should be used (Johnstone, 1979). The sections are usually cut at 6–7 µm, with a slightly reduced rake and a well-cooled block. It may also help if the floating-out bath is slightly hotter than normal; otherwise use water-free (dry) alcohol in the last dehydration step to help avoid lifting of the sections—especially teeth.

Only small pieces of undecalcified bone can be cut with a Ralph knife or tungsten carbide knife. Frozen undecalcified 7–12 µm sections are sometimes used for histochemical purposes. Unembedded undecalcified tissues tend to crumble and shatter when cut; various workers have used adhesives, either on a tape (Ball, 1957; Duthie, 1954; Hart, 1962), as a pressure-sensitive system (Hill and Elde, 1990) or with PVP (McElroy *et al.*, 1993). Cancellous, spongy bone, rather than dense cortical bone, is best suited to frozen sectioning. Tissues should be washed well so that residual acids and fixatives do not interfere with freezing, or corrode the knife.

3.20.4 Wax impregnation

The resulting tissue always remains tough and hard to cut because of the collagen component, despite decalcification; the best method is to embed in a hard wax, nitrocellulose or resin. Formol-saline is often recommended as better than neutral buffered formalin for decalcified tissues. Page *et al.* (1990) give the following protocol.

70% ethanol, or secondary fixation in mercuric chloride-formalin	8 h
90% ethanol	8 h
95% ethanol	24 h
50:50% absolute ethanol/ether	8 h
1% celloidin in ether	16 h
Chloroform	16 h
Hard paraffin wax (m.p. 58°C)	16 h
Two changes of wax under vacuum	16 h

3.20.5 Resin impregnation

Both decalcified and untreated bone can be embedded in acrylic resin, either LR White, or MMA (Emmanual *et al.*, 1987), GMA (Hott and Marie, 1987) or butyl methacrylate. Some workers recommend that bones are defatted with chloroform or acetone after dehydration in absolute alcohol, and also embedded under vacuum to permit uniform polymerization of the resin. The tissue should be returned to absolute alcohol after chloroform treatment to remove this reagent before impregnation with resin. It is particularly important with large specimens to ensure that they are thoroughly dehydrated to avoid problems with polymerization. Resin mixtures are particularly useful for studying bone implants (Murice-Lambert *et al.*, 1989). Isopropanol (propan-2-ol) or ethanol are suitable dehydrants, and a small amount of propan-2-ol in the xylene will prevent disruption of the sections. Some workers dehydrate using terpineol or Euparal essence and mount in Euparal where folds in sections present problems. Sections can otherwise be mounted in resin.

3.21 Lignified tissues

For most herbaceous, woody material with a relatively thin lignified exterior, it is usually sufficient to dissect slices or take them with a hand microtome (Section 4.13), and process them in the normal way after fixation with a suitable botanical fixative, such as CRAF or FAA. For accurate examination of wood sections, however, extensive softening and the expulsion of air from the internal cells is necessary for good infiltration and microtomy. The blocks of wood should be sawn, and then chiselled or planed smooth, not exceeding 10 mm^3. Blocks of wood should be boiled until they become water-logged and sink. Replacement of the hot water for cold between repeated boilings will hasten this step. If the blocks of refractory tissue need to be softened before microtomy, then one of the fluids listed in Section 4.11.1 can be used.

Many of the softer woods can then be sectioned, but harder woods will require further softening. The traditional fluid is 50% hydrofluoric acid, which is *extremely corrosive*, and cannot be used with glassware. Relatively soft woods such as oak, teak and yew should be left to soak for 2–4 days, while much harder types, such as ebony, will require 9–12 days. After soaking, the blocks must be washed free of all residual acid, and stored in 15% glycerol in ethanol for a few days before sectioning. This mixture can also be used to store the softer wood blocks if sectioning is not carried out immediately.

Another method is to reflux the wood blocks in 50% glacial acetic acid in 20 volumes hydrogen peroxide for 1–2 h. When softened, the outer faces of the block will assume a pale or white appearance. The blocks should be washed thoroughly for at least 12 h before sectioning, and both softening methods must not be overdone or the tissue will become macerated. Where maceration is intended, in order to study isolated wood fibres, one of the methods in Section 5.6.1 can be used.

A sliding microtome is used to cut the sections, with the knife set to a 10° horizontal tilt, and up to 10° clearance angle. As with cutting cellulose sections, the block and knife should both be flooded with 70% ethanol. The sections can be stained free-floating in safranin and/or light green, and mounted either as a temporary glycerol jelly or permanent resin mount. Where three sections (transverse, radial and tangential) are mounted under one cover, it is easiest if the minimum amount of resin is applied to the slide and a very small streak also applied to the coverslip. The coverslip should be weighted down while the preparation is drying. Further details are given in Jane (1970).

If the wood blocks are too large to cut with a microtome, or maceration must be avoided, it is possible to cut slices of wood (10 × 10 × 2 mm) with a band saw and embed the slice in resin (Beals and Guard, 1958). The preparation can then be considered as similar to a petrographic specimen, and a thin section prepared in the same way. For suitable details, the reader is referred to Humphries (1992). The wood sections can be stained as usual (Section 6.3.6; 6.4.2), or if it is intended to study unstained sections, the contrast of these specimens can be increased by polishing the upper surface of the specimen with alumina powder (Larson, 1959).

Tissues containing a lot of chlorophyll, such as leaves, may have to be bleached before clearing and mounting (for a discussion see Gardner, 1975). A modified method has been published by Kurth (1978), which is as follows.

1. Leaves are fixed in 95% ethanol overnight or, if dried, soaked in 95% ethanol for 1 h at 50°C.

2. The tannin is removed by bleaching with Stockwell's bleach, which is 1% chromic acid and 1% potassium dichromate in 10% acetic acid, for 1–2 days. The leaves should then be washed in running water for several hours.
3. Stain the tissue in 1% safranin in 50% ethanol for 2 days.
4. Rinse and differentiate in 5% sodium hydroxide for up to 5 weeks, until only the veins remain dark and the other tissues are light pink. Replace the solution with fresh sodium hydroxide each week.
5. Dehydrate from 50% ethanol through to two changes of *t*-butanol (2-methyl propan-2-ol) for 5 min each.
6. Transfer to an equal mixture of 2-methyl propan-2-ol and xylene for 15 min, and mount in a xylene-based resin.

An alternative technique has been published by Rao *et al.* (1980), and a modification suitable for examining thick zoological sections by Perry *et al.* (1975).

3.22 Insect tissues

Insects present a challenge to histologists in the same way as teeth, where a hard outer exoskeleton must be treated for microtomy without destroying the internal soft tissues. Partial infiltration is usually used followed by dissolution of the exocuticle by mineral acids or commercial reagents. For a review of these methods the reader is referred to Haas (1992). A method using Mukerji's or Carnoy's fluid to fix tissues and soften the exoskeleton simultaneously, followed by double embedding, has been used by Sinha (1953). The technique varies from Peterfi's double embedding method (Section 3.16.1) only in that the final block is not hardened in pure chloroform, but is kept in a 17% solution of paraffin wax in chloroform overnight.

Mukerji's fluid

Saturated aqueous picric acid in 90% ethanol	75 ml
10% formalin	25 ml
Concentrated nitric acid	8 ml

This mixture is very similar to alcoholic Bouin's with nitric substituted for the acetic acid. Mix these reagents in the order stated. The addition of 5% mercuric chloride is recommended for prolonged immersion (more than a week) to soften the cuticle. The rapidly acting Carnoy's fluid is replaced by 5% nitric acid in 90% ethanol for 1 week.

For whole mounts of insects and arthropods, the reverse process is carried out: the internal tissues are macerated and cleared, while the exocuticle is softened and prepared for mounting. The organism should be preserved in absolute isopropyl alcohol (propan-2-ol), at which stage it can be stored indefinitely. Prior to mounting, the chitin is softened and the body fluids removed by immediate transfer and heating a number of times in 20% sodium hydroxide. The organism can then be dissected as required in water, dehydrated in propan-2-ol and mounted after passage through a transition medium. Fuller details on preparing insect whole mounts, and mounting specimens dry or in glycerin jelly, can be found in Ives (1984a, b).

3.23 Hair fibres

Before examination hair should be cleaned in a mixture of equal volumes of diethyl ether and ethanol. The sample can then be dried flat between *lightly* weighted filter papers. Hairs should be held in place on the slide with gum tragacanth, and mounted in glycerin jelly or Euparal. Transverse sections may be prepared by the plate method of Ford and Simmens (Syred, 1991). A plate $76 \times 25 \times 0.2$ mm is constructed from shim steel, with a central 0.6–0.8 mm diameter hole. About a dozen fibres are gathered, folded over, and pulled through the hole. A single-edged razor blade is used to cut the sample on either side. The preparation is examined *in situ* once mountant and a coverslip have been applied. If cellulose acetate packing yarn is used to hold the sample in place, this can be dissolved using acetone, and the sample (welded into one mass) permanently mounted in the usual way, rather than within the steel plate.

3.24 Diatom frustules

The siliceous frustules of diatoms are well known as test-objects for correctly setting-up the light microscope (Sanderson, 1990). Before use the samples must be cleaned of organic material and protoplasm. If possible, a pure sample should be collected; diatoms are phototrophic, and can often be scraped off the surface of mud and stones, or else wrung out of weeds. Granular debris, which is unavoidable in collections, can be 'panned' out be swirling in a crystallizing dish. Take *care* with the concentrated acids.

1. Wash the sample in distilled water, centrifuge at 50 *g* for 5 min, decant the supernatant and resuspend in distilled water. Repeat twice.
2. Add concentrated hydrochloric acid dropwise. If calcerous effervescence occurs, leave for 24 h, agitating occasionally. Repeat if the solution is coloured yellow due to iron salts.
3. Wash with distilled water three times, as in (1).

4. Dilute 1/3 volume of diatoms with 2/3 volume of 20% (aq) sulphuric acid. *Care!*
5. Add a few drops of saturated aqueous (8%) potassium permanganate, this generates heat with effervescence. Add further permanganate every 5 min, until the solution remains purple. Agitate by pipetting over 24 h.
6. Gradually add saturated oxalic acid to decolorize. The suspension should go milky, then clear.
7. Wash the sample with distilled water, as in (1), several times, since the frustules will trap chemicals. Examine microscopically: if floc and organic matter are present, add a few drops of 20% sodium hydroxide and centrifuge at 120 g for 15 sec. Decant supernatant and wash twice. This treatment will dissolve the pectin and remove the girdle bands, and should be used with caution.
8. Preserve the sample with a few drops of 1% phenol.

This method has been taken from Hendey (1974). An alternative method, using heat, is described by Ma and Jeffrey (1978).

3.25 Recording tissue processing

Preparing tissues for microscopical examination is often lengthy. The most time-consuming stage is fixing and processing the raw tissue to where preparation may be interrupted and the tissue stored as blocks or sections. In some cases material must be processed from start to finish more or less without interruption. Most laboratories will, therefore, have several specimens at various stages of preparation at a given time. It is easier to keep track of the process of microtechnique if either a whiteboard with dry markers or (better) a pegboard is used to record progress. The identification of each specimen can be recorded on the tops of flat-headed pins, and these moved to each separate processing step as required.

References

Acetarin JD, Carlemalm E, Villiger W. (1986) Development of new Lowicryl® resins for embedding specimens at even lower temperatures. *J. Microsc.* **143**, 81–88.
Altman LG, Schneider BG, Papermaster DS. (1984) Rapid embedding of tissues in Lowicryl K4M for immunoelectron microscopy. *J. Histochem. Cytochem.* **32**, 1217–1223.
Ameele RJ. (1976) A method for the preparation of serial thick sections of plastic-embedded plant tissues. *Stain Technol.* **51**, 17–24.

Anker GCh, Scheers-Dubbeldam K, Noorlander C. (1974) An epoxy resin embedding technique for large objects. *Stain Technol.* **49**, 183–187.

Arnolds WJA. (1978) Orientated embedding of small objects in agar-paraffin, with reference marks for serial section reconstruction. *Stain Technol.* **53**, 287–288.

Ashford AE, Allaway WG, Gubler F, Lennon A, Sleegers J. (1986) Temperature control in Lowicryl K4M and glycol methacrylate during polymerization: is there a low temperature method? *J. Microsc.* **144**, 107–126.

Ball J. (1957) A simple method of defining osteoid in undecalcified sections. *J. Clin. Pathol.* **10**, 281–282.

Beals HO, Guard AT. (1958) An abrasive paper technique for preparing sections of wood for microscopic study. *Stain Technol.* **33**, 103–108.

Bennett HS, Wyrick AD, Lee SW, McNeil Jr JH. (1976) Science and art in preparing plastic for light microscopy, with special reference to glycol methacrylate, glass knives and simple stains. *Stain Technol.* **51**, 71–97.

Brain EB. (1966) *The Preparation of Decalcified Sections.* Thomas, Springfield.

Brain EB. (1974) Processing histological specimens: a rapid method. *Microscopy* **32**, 427–432.

Britten KM, Howarth PH, Roche WR. (1993) Immunohistochemistry on resin sections: a comparison of resin embedding techniques for small mucosal biopsies. *Biotechnic Histochem.* **68**, 271–280.

Buzzell GR. (1975) Double-embedding techniques for light microscope histology. *Stain Technol.* **50**, 285–287.

Causton BE. (1980) The molecular structure of resins and its effect on the epoxy embedding resins. *Proc. R. Microscop. Soc.* **15**, 185–189.

Causton BE, RMS Safety Sub-Committee. (1981) Resins: toxicity, hazards & safe handling. *Proc. R. Microscop. Soc.* **16**, 265–271.

Causton BE. (1988) The hazards associated with embedding resins. *Microsc. Anal.* **3**, 19–21.

Crowley HH, Leichtling BH. (1989) Elimination or reduction of wrinkles in semithin epoxy sections by vacuum drying. *Stain Technol.* **64**, 221–223.

Culling CFA, Allison RT, Barr WT. (1985) *Cellular Pathology Technique*, 4th edn. Butterworths, London.

Drury RAB, Wallington EA. (1980) *Carleton's Histological Technique*, 5th edn. Oxford University Press, Oxford.

Duthie RB. (1954) A simple method for cutting sections of undecalcified bone for subsequent autoradiography and microscopy. *J. Pathol. Bacteriol.* **68**, 296.

Emmanual J, Hornbeck C, Bloebaum RD. (1987) A polymethyl methacrylate method for large specimens of mineralised bone with implants. *Stain Technol.* **62**, 401–410.

Feder N, O'Brien TP. (1968) Plant microtechnique: some principles and new methods. *Am. J. Botany* **55**, 123–142.

Foschini MP, Muzzi L. (1993) A method for decalcification with citric acid. *Biotechnic Histochem.* **68**, 42–45.

Frangioni G, Borgioli G. (1979) Polystyrene embedding: a new method for light and electron microscopy. *Stain Technol.* **54**, 167–176.

Gao K, Godkin JD. (1991) A new method for transfer of PEG-embedded tissue sections to silanated slides for immunocytochemistry. *J. Histochem. Cytochem.* **39**, 537–540.

Gardner RO. (1975) An overview of botanical clearing technique. *Stain Technol.* **50**, 99–105.

Gerrits PO, van Leeuwen MBM, Boon ME, Kok LP. (1987) Floating on a water bath and mounting glycol methacrylate and hydroxypropyl methacrylate sections influence final dimensions. *J. Microsc.* **145**, 107–113.

Glauert AM. (1991) Epoxy resins: an update on their selection and use. *Microsc. Anal.* **25**, 15–20.

Gordon KC. (1990) Tissue processing. In *Theory and Practice of Histological Techniques*, 3rd edn (eds JD Bancroft and A Stevens). Churchill Livingstone, Edinburgh, pp. 43–59.

Graham ET. (1982) Improved diethylene glycol distearate embedding wax. *Stain Technol.* **57**, 39–43.

Gray P. (1954) *The Microtomist's Formulary and Guide.* Blakiston, New York.

Guyer MF. (1953) *Animal Micrology*, 6th edn. University of Chicago Press, Chicago.

Haas F. (1992) Serial sectioning of insects with hard exoskeleton by dissolution of the exocuticle. *Biotechnic Histochem.* **67**, 50–54.

Hart P. (1962) A support backing for the cutting of friable sections. *J. Med. Lab. Technol.* **19**, 115–116.

Hayat MA. (1989) *Principles and Techniques of Electron Microscopy: Biological Applications*, 3rd edn. Macmillan, Basingstoke.

Hemenway AF. (1930) Some new methods and combinations in plant microtechnique. *Science* **72**, 251–252.

Hendey NI. (1974) The permanganate method for cleaning freshly-gathered diatoms. *Microscopy* **32**, 423–426.

Hernández Mariné MC. (1992) A simple way to encapsulate small samples for processing in TEM. *J. Microsc.* **168**, 203–206.

Hilger HH, Medan D. (1987) A simple method for exact alignment of small paraffin embedded specimens to the cutting plane. *Stain Technol.* **62**, 282–283.

Hill EL, Elde R. (1990) An improved method for preparing cryostat sections of undecalcified bone for multiple uses. *J. Histochem. Cytochem.* **38**, 443–448.

Hillmer S, Joachim S, Robinson DG. (1991) Rapid polymerization of LR White for immunocytochemistry. *Histochemistry* **95**, 315–318.

Horobin RW. (1989) *Understanding of Staining of Water-miscible Resin Sections.* DataScope Services, University of Sheffield.

Hott M, Marie PJ. (1987) Glycol methacrylate as an embedding medium for bone. *Stain Technol.* **62**, 51–57.

Humphries DW. (1992) *The Preparation of Thin Sections of Rocks, Minerals, and Ceramics.* Royal Microscopical Society Handbook 24, Oxford University Press, Oxford.

Ives E. (1984a) Whole mounts of insects. *Microscopy* **35**, 45–51.

Ives E. (1984b) Further notes on whole mounts of insects. *Microscopy* **35**, 115–116.

Jane FW. (1970) *The Structure of Wood*, 2nd edn (revised by K Wilson, DJB White). A&C Black, London.

Janes RB. (1979) A review of three resin processing techniques applicable to light microscopy. *Med. Lab. Sci.* **36**, 249–267.

Janisch R. (1974) Orientated embedding of single-cell organisms. *Stain Technol.* **49**, 157–160.

Johannessen JV. (1977) Use of paraffin material for electron microscopy. *Pathol. Annu.* **12**, 189–224.

Johnstone JJA. (1979) The routine sectioning of undecalcified bone for cytochemical studies. *Histochem. J.* **11**, 359–365.

Kent AP. (1991) The routine use of polyester wax for immunohistochemistry. *Microsc. Anal.* **24**, 37.

Kiernan JA. (1990) *Histological & Histochemical Methods: Theory & Practice*, 2nd edn. Pergamon Press, Oxford.

Klosen P, Maessen X, de Aguilar PvdB. (1993) PEG embedding for immunocytochemistry: application to the analysis of immunoreactivity loss during histological processing. *J. Histochem. Cytochem.* **41**, 455–463.

Kurth E. (1978) A modified method for clearing leaves. *Stain Technol.* **53**, 291–293.

Lang AG. (1937) The use of *n*-butyl alcohol in the paraffin method. *Stain Technol.* **12**, 113–117.

Larson PR. (1959) Preparation of small wood blocks for photomicrography. *Stain Technol.* **34**, 155–156.

Lillie RD, Fullmer HM. (1976) *Histopathological Technique and Practical Histochemistry*, 4th edn. McGraw-Hill, New York.

Litwin JA. (1985) Light microscopic histochemistry on plastic sections. *Prog. Histochem. Cytochem.* **16**, 1–84.

McElroy HH, Shih M-S, Parfitt AM. (1993) Producing frozen sections of calcified bone. *Biotechnic Histochem.* **68**, 50–55.

Ma JCW, Jeffrey LM. (1978) Description and comparison of a new cleaning method of diatom frustules for light and electron microscope studies. *J. Microsc.* **112**, 235–238.

Miller RT, Groothuis CL. (1991) Multitumor 'sausage' blocks in immunohistochemistry. *Am. J. Clin. Pathol.* **96**, 228–232.

Murgatroyd LB. (1976) The preparation of thin sections from glycol methacrylate embedded tissue using a standard rotary microtome. *Med. Lab. Sci.* **33**, 67–71.

Murice-Lambert E, Banford AB, Folger RL. (1989) Histological preparation of implanted biomaterials for light-microscopic evaluation of the implant-tissue interaction. *Stain Technol.* **64**, 19–24.

Murray GI. (1988) Is wax on the wane? *J. Pathol.* **156**, 187–188.

Newman GR. (1987) The use and abuse of LR White. *Histochem. J.* **19**, 118–120.

Newman GR, Hobot JA. (1987) Modern acrylics for post-embedding immunostaining techniques. *J. Histochem. Cytochem.* **35**, 971–981.

Nuttall DS. (1986) Polymerisation of LR Gold resin using white light. *Med. Lab. Sci.* **43**, 289–291.

Page K, Stevens A, Lowe J, Bancroft JD. (1990) Bone. In *Theory and Practice of Histological Techniques*, 3rd edn (eds JD Bancroft and A Stevens). Churchill Livingstone, Edinburgh. pp. 309–341.

Perry LJ, Harbison RM, Lumb R. (1975) The use of Herr four-and-a-half clearing fluid for the rapid microscopic examination of thick sections of normal and neoplastic tissues. *Stain Technol.* **50**, 47–50.

Postek MT. (1978) Mounting cleared botanical preparations. *Stain Technol.* **53**, 178–179.

Prentø P. (1985) A reliable and simple method for orientated epoxy embedding of tissue sections and strips using horizontal polyethylene BEEM capsules. *Stain Technol.* **60**, 120–122.

Rao VS, Shenoy KN, Inamdar JA. (1980) Clearing and staining technique for leaf architectural studies. *Microscop. Acta* **83**, 307–310.

Redmond BL, Bob C. (1984) A fixation/dehydration/infiltration apparatus that minimises human exposure to harmful chemicals. *J. Electron Microsc. Tech.* **1**, 97–98.

Richards PR. (1980) A technique for obtaining ribbons of epoxy and other plastic sections for light microscope histology. *J. Microsc.* **122**, 213–216.

Ridgway RL, Chestnut MH. (1984) Processing small tissue specimens in acrylic resins for ultramicrotomy: improved handling and orientation. *J. Electron Microsc. Tech.* **1**, 205–206.

Roberts DMcL, Warren A. (1987) An inexpensive apparatus for automatic continuous dehydration. *Stain Technol.* **62**, 211–215.

Rostgaard J, Buchmann B. (1974) Problems in ultraviolet polymerisation of embedding media for elecron microscopy. *J. Microsc.* **102**, 187–193.

Sanderson JB. (1990) The measurement of three light microscope test diatoms by scanning electron microscopy. *Proc. R. Microscop. Soc.* **25**, 195–203.

Scala C, Cenacchi G, Ferrari C, Pasquinelli G, Preda P, Manara GC. (1992) A new acrylic resin formulation: a useful tool for histological, ultrastructural and immunocytochemical investigations. *J. Histochem. Cytochem.* **40**, 1799–1804.

Sene F deM. (1991) Reference markers in serial sections. *Biotechnic Histochem.* **136**, 136–138.

Sims B. (1974) A simple method of preparing 1–2 µm sections of large tissue blocks using glycol methacrylate. *J. Microsc.* **101**, 223–227.

Sinha RN. (1953) Sectioning insects with sclerotized cuticle. *Stain Technol.* **28**, 249–253.

Smith M, Croft S. (1991) Embedding and thin section preparation. In *Electron Microscopy in Biology* (ed. JR Harris). Oxford University Press, Oxford, pp. 17–37.

Sommer JR, Taylor I, Scherer B. (1979) Wrinkle-free thick sections of tissues embedded in hard plastics. *Stain Technol.* **54**, 106–107.

Steedman HF. (1960) *Section Cutting in Microscopy.* Blackwells, Oxford.

Stevens A, Germain J. (1990) Resin embedding media. In *Theory and Practice of Histological Techniques*, 3rd edn (eds JD Bancroft and A Stevens). Churchill Livingstone, Edinburgh. pp. 497–507.

Syred A. (1991) Microscopy of mammalian hair. *Microsc. Anal.* **24**, 23–25.

Tobler M, Freiburghaus AU. (1990) Occupational risks of (meth)acrylate compounds in embedding media for electron microscopy. *J. Microsc.* **160**, 291–298.

4 Microtomy

The various types of microtome and knife available, as well as the mechanics of keeping a good knife, are described before the methods for cutting good quality thin paraffin wax and resin sections. This is in order that the mechanics which determine particular procedures are made clear.

Above all, it is important to keep a well-sharpened knife. The importance of this cannot be over-stated: it is better to keep a knife in good condition and hone or strop it a little at a time to preserve a good keen edge than to allow a good knife edge gradually to deteriorate without frequent attention. A bad knife edge is far more likely than anything else to lead to inconsistencies, poor quality sections and the need to refer to the fault-diagnosis tables (see *Tables 4.3* and *4.4*).

4.1 Types of microtome

4.1.1 Hand microtome

The hand microtome for freehand sectioning is rarely used. It is limited to cutting hardened tissues, mainly of botanical origin, and is described in Section 4.13.

4.1.2 Cambridge rocking microtome

This classical instrument was developed in 1885, and revolutionized specimen preparation methods (*Figure 4.1*). The microtome is mechanically very simple and has few moving parts: the captive nut and screw which determines section thickness, and the rocking arm. The rotary rocker is, therefore, often used in cryostats where a minimum of moving parts are exposed to freezing.

The tissue is mounted onto cylindrical chucks which are held in the rocking arm by a screw clamp; the section advance is from 2 to 25 μm in 1 μm steps. The stationary knife holder will accept most profiles, and the

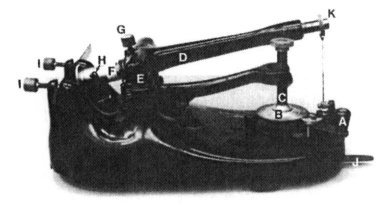

Figure 4.1:   The Cambridge rocking microtome. The handle (A) operates the captive nut (B) on the thread (C), which determines the advance of the rocking arm (D), which rests on two fulcra (E). The specimen chuck (F) is secured on the rocking arm by the screw clamp (G). The orientation of the block to the knife can be altered within limits by the eccentric lever (H) on the chuck. The Heiffor knife illustrated is secured by the screw clamps (I). The lever (J) at the base of the instrument click-stops into three positions, which will alter the radius of arc of the rocking arm, to suit the size of the block, and the tension of the rocking stroke may be adjusted by turning the knob (K) attached to the catgut cord (photograph courtesy of Mr Terry Cooper).

knife angle can be altered within limits by two screw clamps at the front of the instrument. Rocking microtomes cut sections which are very slightly curved. Moreover, the block size taken by a rocking microtome is limited to 20 × 25 mm, and it is not possible to move the knife holder laterally as with other types of microtome. The 'rocker' is a lightweight machine, and as such is not suited to cutting hard tissues, unlike a rotary or sliding microtome. Because of the microtome's lightness, and the tendency of the section advance to jerk, it may be an advantage to operate the instrument on a rubber anti-vibration mat.

4.1.3 Rotary microtomes

This type of instrument is widely used, and is also called the Minot microtome (*Figure 4.2*). The knife is stationary, and the block is held in a ball joint, permitting it to be orientated to the knife edge. Most instruments have a retractable arm that moves away from the block on the upstroke, and the handwheel may be locked with the arm in this position. Where a microtome will retract the specimen from the knife edge on the return stroke to avoid fouling the surface of the block against the back of the knife edge, it is called a double-pass instrument. Simpler models, in which this is not the case, are referred to as single-pass instruments. The micrometer feed mechanism is based on a gear-train, and is both accurate and hard-wearing; the section thickness can be set from 1 to 25 μm. Larger blocks can be cut on this microtome, and the sections are flat, since the cutting

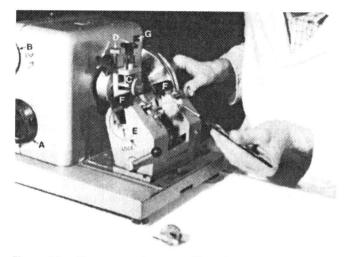

Figure 4.2:   The rotary microtome. The micrometer feed (A) can be seen on the lower left side of the picture, and the specimen arm retraction on the upper left (B). The chuck (C) can be orientated by means of the screw clamps (D). The clearance angle of the knife can be set by rotation within the knife holder (E), which slides and may be locked in the desired position. Two magnetic knife guards (F) can be seen in position, and this model has a section counter in the top right-hand corner (G) (photograph courtesy of Dr Savile Bradbury).

arm does not describe an arc. This instrument is heavier than the rocking microtome, and can easily cut wax, celloidin and resin sections.

4.1.4 Base-sledge and sliding microtomes

These models have a greater mass than rotary microtomes, and are suitable for cutting celloidin and resin sections. They also allow the knife edge to be set obliquely rather than perpendicular to the block face, and this can be useful when sectioning hard tissue where a lower effective cutting angle is required (Section 4.3.1). In the heavier base-sledge (*Figure 4.3*) the knife is held static with the specimen held on a runner, while the arrangement is reversed in the sliding microtome (*Figure 4.4*). It is important to keep the rail clean and lightly oiled, to ensure smooth sectioning with either type. The section thickness can be set from 1 to 25 µm; the specimen is advanced either by a manual handwheel, or automatically by a lever mechanism operated as the specimen approaches the knife. With the latter it is possible to cut sections of a multiple of the set thickness by clocking half strokes before taking a cut.

The sliding microtome is lighter and cheaper than the base-sledge. In some models the specimen holder rises vertically as the tissue advances for the next section, while in others the specimen holder rises on an inclined plane towards the knife. In this latter case, care should be taken that the block is not so large that it will not have sufficient room to section completely. It is possible to cut serial sections on a base-sledge or sliding

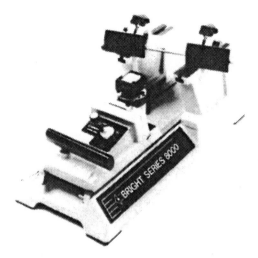

Figure 4.3: The base-sledge microtome. The section thickness gauge and advance mechanism may be seen on the sledge to the front. The sprung block holder shown takes standard plastic cassettes. In this type of microtome the block, with its holder and advance mechanism, is moved with respect to a fixed knife (photograph courtesy of the Bright Instrument Co.).

microtome, particularly if a smear of low-melting point wax is applied to the top face of the block, but serial sections are best cut on a rotary microtome.

4.1.5 Freezing microtome

This instrument is useful for cutting frozen sections with the minimum of equipment, but has largely been superseded by the cryostat. It clamps to the bench and has a small swinging knife with a bevel angle of about 40°, which is set at a cutting angle of about 15° or more. Because the resulting rake angle is small, the instrument is not suited to cutting uniform thin sections, and distortion may occur. The action of the swinging knife permits only small blocks to be cut; producing ribbons of serial sections is impossible. The knife and stage are cooled by compressed liquid carbon dioxide released in bursts, or an electric cooling stage operating on the Peltier effect may be used. The electrical stage will rapidly freeze specimens down to –50°C in a few seconds; it is illustrated, with a good account of its action, in Bancroft (1967). When using a carbon dioxide cylinder, check whether it has to be used in the upright or inverted position: if it is incorrectly used, only gas will emerge, and this is ineffective for freezing tissue blocks. Check that the liquid carbon dioxide is flowing freely to the stage, and freeze the tissue in bursts until the frost line has reached the top of the block. If the knife is cooled to roughly the same temperature as the block, then not only will it be easier to cut thin sections, but these will

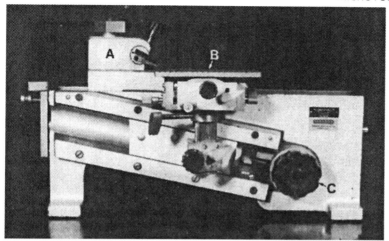

Figure 4.4:   The sliding microtome. Side view of the sliding microtome. The sliding knife is held on a sledge (A), while the stage (B) advances up the incline by a rachet mechanism, either by the handwheel (C), or automatically by movement of the knife (photograph courtesy of Dr Savile Bradbury).

not stick to the knife, and so can be removed with a paintbrush. Cut sections at 6–8 μm, and fatty sections at 10–15 μm.

4.1.6 Automated microtomes

Laboratories have used automated cryostats for a number of years, and research has recently been published (Vincent, 1991) on the computer control of rotary microtomes for cutting wax and resin sections.

4.2 Clamps and chucks

The most common type of clamp is the screw clamp which holds the chuck in a recess in the microtome arm, or specimen plate. A spring-loaded vice type is particularly useful for the routine sectioning of large quantities of blocks where the block must be changed over and faced-off rapidly. In the converse situation, where orientation is paramount, a ball-joint or Naples clamp (which moves multilaterally) allows the block to be orientated precisely.

Holders can be of various designs (*Figure 4.5*), from simple wooden blocks and cylinders or stubs with a series of concentric or square cut ridges, to large brass platforms. For routine work, the tissue is often contained in a coloured plastic cassette which accepts a metal or plastic snap-on lid. The tissue, thus boxed, is processed and embedded with the plastic cassette serving as a platform to lock into a sprung-loaded vice. A

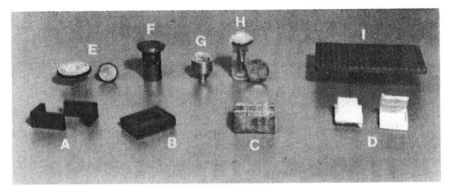

Figure 4.5: Clamps, holders and Leuckhart pieces. In the front row two Leuckhart 'L' pieces are shown (A), and placed together (B); this is usually done on a separate baseplate. A wooden blockholder (C), and plastic cassettes (D) are also shown. The cast block is on the left and the empty cassette on the right. In the back row are two cryostat chucks (E) with rubber insulating rings to prevent coldburns whilst handling. The Cambridge rocking microtome chuck is shown (F). A turned aluminium chuck is shown with a resin block (G), and a metal chuck (with Bijou bottle as holder) for wax blocks (H). The brass stage (I) is suitable for holding fixed frozen specimens on a sliding microtome.

flat face ensures that the block is faced-off and the sections cut with the minimum of tissue or time wasted. A design for a miniature vice has been published by Godkin and Knight (1975) for use where the specimen block is too small to be held in a standard vice, although this should not present problems with the plastic embedding cassettes in regular use.

4.3 Types of knives

There are four different profiles of microtome knife: A, BL, C and D, illustrated in *Figure 4.6*. The biconcave (BL) profile may also be called the Heiffor knife, while the other types are called Jung knives. These knives range in length from 90 mm (like the Heiffor) to 350 mm. The Heiffor knives tend to have an integral handle, while the Jung types are supplied with detachable handles that can be screwed in, when required, for sharpening.

The wedge (C) or 'universal' knife is the most common. It is suitable for cutting wax, celloidin, resin and frozen sections and is easier to use than other types. The bevel angle is usually 31°. The planoconcave type (A) should be used with the concave face trailing away from and the plane face facing the block; it is principally used for wax and celloidin sections, and will take a keener bevel angle than the wedge, but is less robust for hard tissues than either the wedge or tool edge profiles.

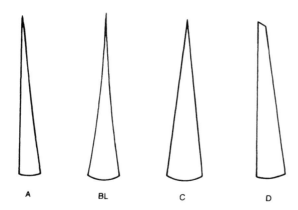

A   BL   C   D

Figure 4.6:   Knife profiles. The 'A' profile is planoconcave, and is used with the concave edge trailing. The 'BL' is biconcave (hollow-ground), while the 'C' or wedge profile is most commonly used. The massive 'D' profile with a tool edge is used for very hard materials, and may be sintered tungsten carbide.

The biconcave hollow-ground (BL or Heiffor type) knife is lighter than either of the above profiles, but will accept a very small cutting angle and will cut keenly all but the hardest tissue. These types must be sharpened manually without the use of a knife back. Heiffor knives are supplied with a cutting angle of either 17° for cutting soft, or 22° for cutting hard, tissues. The shallow rake angle of the tool edge (D) makes it unsuited to routine sectioning of soft materials, but ideal for very hard material, such as wood and undecalcified bone. These knives are difficult to resharpen.

The Heiffor knife is not usually sharpened with a knife back, or honing bevel, although some workers use a spring-on tubular type of back. Without a knife back, metal is removed from both the facet and back of the knife during sharpening; this reduces the cutting angle, necessitating alteration when inserted into the microtome, and periodic re-grinding of the correct cutting angle onto the knife. This does not occur when a knife back is used, because metal is removed from the facets alone, and the cutting angle remains constant.

Most microtome knives are made from steel; a good quality carbon or tool steel is tempered for one third in from the blade edge, the hardness being 400–900 on the Vickers hardness scale. Cutting with a temper of 900 is best, but the tip is more brittle, and more prone to damage from chipping on hard inclusions, particularly with a small cutting angle ground onto the knife. However, if the knife temper is too soft, then the edge will be rapidly dulled, and so a compromise must be sought between knife temper and cutting angle. Ideally, the knife edge should be tempered as hard as is practicable, with the mass of the knife back providing a softer 'elastic' support to help preserve the edge of the knife.

Sintered tungsten carbide knives provide a tougher, harder blade than steel at 950–1800 hardness. The tungsten carbide is brazed onto a steel body to produce a composite knife. Stellite composite knives, of hardness 400–600, are also available; which do not corrode or chip easily, are resistant to changes in temper when being reground, and are particularly useful for cutting celloidin sections. Tungsten knives with a 35–40° angle should be used to cut GMA blocks, and those of 45–50° to cut undecalcified bone embedded in MMA. Diamond knives are suited for cutting epoxy resins, although glass electron microscopy knives will suffice. Ralph knives are glass knives with an edge parallel to one surface of the glass, instead of across it as for electron microscopy.

4.3.1 Important knife angles and bevels

The cutting edge is a separate facet ground, irrespective of the knife profile, at a known angle with the knife back in place, and not extending more than 1 mm. Too great a bevel presents a larger cutting face to the tissue, with a consequent increase in friction. A separate cutting facet is not present in cryostat knives, to allow the anti-roll plate to lie flat. The bevel of a knife serves the following three functions.

(i)   To reduce the need for sharpening, and removing large quantities of metal to do this.

(ii) To provide a robust edge for cutting.

(iii) To reduce the friction during cutting.

The greater the angle of rake, the easier it is to cut sections (*Figure 4.7*). This angle can only be increased at the expense of the cutting and clearance angles, which may be only a few degrees. The clearance, or tilt, angle of 2–4° allows for the return stroke, without friction damage to the block surface. Suitable cutting angles are small, allowing greater rake and sharper edges. Larger angles, although less efficient, preserve the geometry of the blade from damage. The nomogram (see *Figure 4.18*) can be used by the beginner to set the correct tilt and clearance angles in the microtome. While reduction of the knife slope from the normal reduces the cutting angle, ribboning is prevented and more tissue is in contact with the knife (*Figure 4.8*). A bevel or cutting angle of 17–23° is the best for paraffin work. Angles can be measured with tinplate templates, cut with sharp tinsnips. A more acute edge is required to cut paraffin than resin media. The bevel or facet angle can also be measured by the methods of Powell and Murgatroyd (1970).

Most sectioning is carried out with the knife edge fixed in the vertical plane perpendicular to the axis of travel. If the knife is rotated, or slanted, from the perpendicular axis (particularly when fixed in the horizontal plane as on a sliding microtome) then the slope angle, and hence the *effective* cutting angle, can be reduced. This advantage is gained at a price. A greater width of knife is used to cut the tissue with a shearing cut, which will cause greater friction, compression and possible tearing of soft inhomogenous tissue. It is not possible to produce ribbons with a knife edge offset from the perpendicular axis of travel. However, an obliquely set knife is sometimes useful when cutting hard tissues: in this case the knife edge

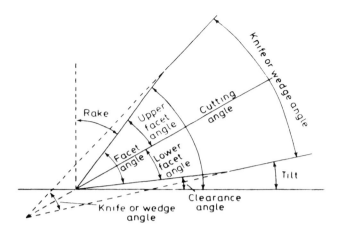

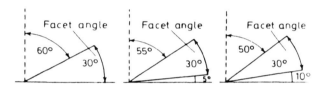

Figure 4.7: Important knife angles. The knife or wedge angle may variously be called the bevel angle. The facet angle may also be termed the cutting angle. Here the cutting angle is the sum of the facet and clearance angle. Note the difference between the clearance and the tilt angles (Gray, 1972).

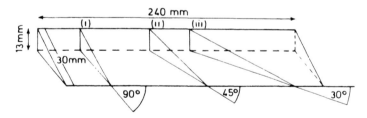

Figure 4.8: The sloping knife. When the knife on a base-sledge or sliding microtome is set obliquely (sloped) from a cutting axis perpendicular to the knife edge, the cutting angle is effectively reduced (Gray, 1972).

is preserved because it does not hit the tissue head-on; the propensity for tearing the tissue out of its block is reduced, yet compression due to the shearing cut is likely to be nearly normal.

4.3.2 Facets

The smaller the facet width, the less the section is distorted by friction. The maximum should be 1 mm, and ideally two or more facets should be superimposed upon the knife bevel. The front facet can then be fine honed to produce a sharp edge, while the rear facet is left sufficiently rugged not to ruin the section, but to reduce frictional contact with it as the section passes to the back of the knife. When the small front facet is polished smooth, a microcrystalline Beilby layer forms from surface flow due to hard smooth abrasion under pressure. The frictional resistance of this layer is high, and has a high affinity for paraffin wax. Superimposing two or more facets on the knife bevel ensures not only that the section will pass relatively unhindered onto the larger, rougher, rear facet, but that less metal must be removed each time the knife is sharpened, and the front facet can be kept to a minimum which can be very quickly stropped.

Highly polished surfaces can be improved by etching the metal, and the affinity of wax for the knife surface can be reduced by coating the knife. The knife may be etched for 2–60 sec in 0.1 M aqueous nitric acid (Collins, 1969) or the following solution (Gray, 1972).

Picric acid (saturated aqueous—1.4%)	330 ml
95% alcohol	170 ml
Teepol (wetting agent)	10 ml
Distilled water	490 ml

4.3.3 Care of knives

Knives should be handled with care and transported in the custom-supplied box sealed with tape. Do not attempt instinctively to catch a falling knife!

Poor knife quality, fixation and embedding are the most commonly encountered avoidable factors that produce artifacts in sections. Artifacts due to fixation and embedding can be rigorously controlled, but the quality and use of the knife for microtomy is very much an operator-dependent variable. A well-kept knife that will cut consistently good sections is beyond price, but given care is not difficult to achieve. A new knife should be checked for the final facet angle by measuring the back and width of each side. The faces (width) and back of the knife should be checked for straightness on an engineer's surface plate or with a steel rule. If the faces are not straight, the facet width may differ and lead to section distortion.

Cryostat knives should be allowed to dry and be lightly oiled between uses to avoid rusting. Some authorities advocate stropping between uses, as ice crystals rapidly blunt the edge. Others prefer to regrind the knife periodically: the argument being that stropping introduces a bevel on the knife edge which does not allow the anti-roll plate to lie flat against the angle of the knife.

4.3.4 Disposable blades

Disposable blades are coming into widespread use, and for all but the hardest or most friable tissue have advantages over steel knives. They are cheap if used wisely, do not require sharpening, and have a more reproducible and reliable edge than a hand-sharpened knife. There is less scoring, and compression is reduced due to the small cutting angle of the blade. Disposable knives cool down quickly for cryotomy, and rusting or sterilization worries are avoided.

It pays to mark one area of the blade with indelible pen, and use this for trimming the block. The remaining sharp area can then be used sequentially to the most economic effect without the need to change blades too often. If the disposable blade is tightened too much into its holder by use of the allen screws, it will tension under load, and can cause chattering of the block. Chattering can be avoided by using a lower cutting speed, or softening the tissue with water or one of the agents listed in Section 4.11.1. Magnetic blades are popular (e.g. the Bright Magnacut) for cryostats. Since there is no need for a blade clamp, the anti-roll plate lies flat against the blade without obstruction. If a screw holder is used, there is always a slight lip edge on the front face of the upper clamp of the holder which can obstruct the thin section coming off the blade. Teflon-coated blades and matching coated holders are available to reduce this problem in cutting frozen sections. With the magnetic type of holder, the wider upper surface of the blade serves as the pick-up area over which the anti-roll plate lies.

4.3.5 Glass and diamond knives

Glass knives. Disposable glass knives were first introduced in 1950 for cutting ultra-thin electron microscopy sections. The usable edge is short, extending for only 60% of the thickness of the glass. They perform better than the conventional steel-edged knife for cutting semi-thin plastic sections of less than 2 µm; knife imperfections from a steel blade occur rapidly, and result in scratched and marred sections. For good cytological detail, sections of the order of 0.2 µm thick are best.

The 'Ralph' knife (Bennett *et al.*, 1976) has a longer edge than the conventional 6.5 mm of the electron microscopy knife, being broken along the face rather than the thickness of the glass strip. The edge is usually 25 mm long, but can be up to 40 mm in length. It is also possible to break 'Ralph' knives from microscope slides (Semba, 1979). The original account by Bennett *et al.* (1976) gives instructions for breaking Ralph knives manually, although there are several histo-knife breakers now on the market. Details of a home-made knife breaker are given by Butler (1979) and the commercial models are described by Reid and Beesley (1991).

The cutting edge of the knife is formed by the upturn of the fracture across the thickness of the glass to the plane face opposite the initial score when the knife is made. This is done by breaking the glass at the site of a score over a fulcrum. It is important to break the glass with the right amount of pressure. If the upturn is too acute, as a result of insufficient pressure, the result is a fragile knife, which will soon break. Too much pressure will provide no cutting edge worth speaking of, with the break being perpendicular to the score over most of the thickness of the glass. On the other hand if the pressure is applied unevenly, then the knife edge will also be uneven, with more flaws along the edge. The cutting angle of Ralph knives is much more variable than those used for ultra-thin sectioning, ranging from 12 to 58°. Isotropic resins, unlike crystalline wax mixtures, will not cut well with knife angles of less than 35°; nevertheless, knives with small cutting angles are more durable than those with larger angles, and cause less compression.

The completed Ralph knife can be mounted with dental wax onto an old steel knife which is used as a holder, although a clamp for the rotary microtome has been described by Szczesny (1978). The clearance angle is usually quoted as 15° for paraffin and 4° for resin sections (Helander, 1984). The Ralph knife can also be used instead of a razor-blade on the Vibratome to section thick histological tissues (Johansson, 1983), and in a cryostat with a special anti-roll plate (Richards, 1984).

Diamond knives. Commercial histo-knives are manufactured by Diatome and DDK with a 45° angle specifically for cutting resin or cryo-sections from 0.2 to 5 μm thick. The usable edge is only 4 mm wide, so that the advantage of the wide edge of the Ralph knife is lost. The advantages are: a sharper knife, thinner sections, reduced preparation time and repeated use of the edge. Despite its extreme initial cost, and the ease with which it can be damaged, a diamond edge is much more tolerant than glass of blocks of varying degrees of hardness, does not have to be replaced, and collecting serial sections is easier. Debris which is allowed to dry onto the knife is extremely difficult to remove, and the knife should be cleaned while still wet. Use pith or a polystyrene rod and ethanol. Solvents such as acetone should not be used since they can dissolve the cement holding the diamond in place.

4.4 Cryotomy

4.4.1 Cold knife methods

The sliding microtome is used to cut serial sections of fixed tissue, which has been treated thus to stabilize soluble or diffusible substances. It is easier and cheaper to use than the cryostat, but only cuts sections which are thicker than 20 μm, while the cryostat has been developed for cutting fresh tissue sections. Fixatives based on aldehydes or picric acid are best. Those containing mercury or dichromate ions are to be avoided, as they tend to make the tissue brittle, while alcohol fixatives raise the freezing point of the tissue, making it difficult or impossible to freeze evenly. Bancroft (1990) recommends the use of formol-calcium.

1. Fix tissue in 10% formol-calcium for 18 h.
2. Wash tissue in running tap water overnight.

3. Transfer to gelatin mixture at 37°C for 6 h.
4. Transfer to fresh gelatin; embed and cool in the refrigerator at 4°C.
5. Trim the block and harden in 10% formol calcium overnight at 4°C.
6. Store the block in fixative or the storage medium in Section 3.13.

For hydrolytic enzymes, the tissue can be fixed as above, followed by a tap water wash for 10 min. The tissue is then blotted dry and embedded in cold gum sucrose at 4°C. The tissue is frozen slowly to –10°C to prevent damage by ice expansion.

The sliding microtome uses a biconcave or wedge profile knife cooled by dry ice, or compressed carbon dioxide. The stage of the microtome should be precooled for 10 min or so in dry ice. The tissue may be mounted directly into 30% sucrose or embedding compound and attached to the precooled stage with distilled water or 30% sucrose. Dry ice, crushed with the mass of the brass stage, should be heaped around the tissue and stage to keep the whole cooled. A paper 'fence' can be constructed to retain the crushed dry ice. Care should be taken to ensure that particles of dry ice do not impinge upon the edge of the blade as it passes over the block.

Some workers prefer to cool the knife in the freezer or refrigerator before use, and keep it cooled periodically using crushed dry ice or carbon dioxide. Others use a warmer knife, particularly if the tissue is well-fixed. The sections are held onto the surface of the knife as they are cut, to prevent curling, and are removed into warm or cold buffer prior to free-floating, staining or mounting onto slides. Excess moisture should be wiped from the front and rear surfaces of the knife with a well-washed lint-free cloth once the section has been removed, and before it passes back over the surface of the block. This ensures that the moisture which collects on the blade does not freeze on the return stroke and so score the surface of the next section.

4.4.2 Cryostats

Most cryostats are placed in a cold chamber, although the latest models merely cool the arm, tissue holder and knife assembly. An anti-roll plate or bar is provided to prevent the sections curling as they are cut. The cryostat differs from the cold knife inasmuch as the knife, tissue and cabinet are within the same temperature range (–10 to –26°C) (*Figure 4.9*).

4.5 Freezing

Where fixed frozen sections are to be cut, it is sufficient to cool the tissue relatively slowly using dry ice (–70°C) or an aerosol spray (–50°C). However, slow cooling is insufficient for cryotomy of fresh tissue, as damage arises from the intercellular nucleation and growth of ice crystals. Not only

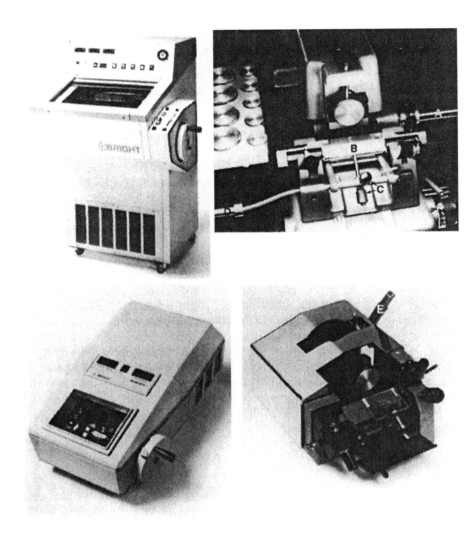

Figure 4.9:   The cryostat. The Bright cryostat (top, left). The optional motorized control unit can be seen on the right by the hand-wheel. A view inside the freezer cabinet (top, right). The hand-wheel link (A) is to the right of the picture. The anti-roll plate (B) and adjusting screws (C) are in the centre, while the link to retract the anti-roll plate (D) is seen to the left. The Starlet minature microtome is shown (bottom, left), with the internal mechanism (bottom, right). The lever (E) provides an alternative control to the hand-wheel. In this picture the white tape on the anti-roll plate, providing clearance for sections to pass off the knife, can be clearly seen (photographs courtesy of the Bright Instrument Co).

are tissues disrupted, and labile components lost through slow freezing, but the removal of cell water into the intercellular space alters the salt concentration in the tissue. If this state of affairs continues too long, the freezing point is raised to such an extent that not even liquid nitrogen will freeze the tissue. Aerosol sprays, in particular, do not work well with muscle, which is especially prone to ice crystal damage.

Cell suspensions can be protected by 30% glycerol or 10% dimethyl sulphoxide (DMSO), but rapid freezing is the only effective answer for protecting tissue. Mild pre-fixation with formalin can help, but most freezing artifacts are not visible at the light microscope level in well-prepared tissue. The tissue should be no more than about 5 mm^3, and mounted on a pre-cooled cork mat or metal chuck with water, 20% sucrose or a commercial embedding compound (e.g. Tissue-Tek or Cryo-M-Bed) of polyvinyl alcohol and ethylene glycol. Tissues are best frozen with either liquid nitrogen (–196°C), Freon 12 or isopentane cooled in a bath of liquid nitrogen (–150°C). The quenching rate of isopentane is quicker, since a microlayer of liquid nitrogen boils off as it comes into contact with the still warm tissue. This layer retards effective freezing.

4.5.1 Embedding

Fixed tissues are more difficult to prepare for cryotomy, especially if sections thicker than 10 μm are required. Embedding medium can be used to infiltrate the specimens, as well as mounting them on the chuck for cryotomy. One report (Ishii *et al.*, 1990) recommends using three containers of proprietary embedding compound, about 15–30 times the specimen volume, and rotating these in the same way as is done when infiltrating with wax. Fixed specimens, no more than 5 mm thick, are infiltrated for 5, 4 and 15 h at room temperature, and are cut at –5°C once frozen. The authors report good results for Sudan black staining of fat cells, improved thin sectioning and less drying out of blocks during sectioning or storage. Other workers (Barthel and Raymond, 1990) use a sucrose–embedding compound mixture to support limp tissues for thin sectioning, while yet others recommend carboxy-methyl cellulose gel for the same purpose.

If the tissue is cut too thickly (greater than 2 μm) below –70°C, then chattering of the block will occur, and the edge of the knife will become rapidly dulled and blunted. Tissues snap-frozen in liquid nitrogen should be left in the cryostat to warm up for 30 min to 1 h before cutting, depending upon the size of tissue. Tissues that have remained too long in the freezing mixture may become loose, or detach from the metal stub on starting to cut. In this case, the tissue block should be carefully trimmed at the cryostat cabinet temperature of –20°C, and refrozen onto the pre-cooled stub or chuck at this temperature. In this way the differential rates of thermal expansion, which cause detachment between block and chuck, are avoided.

4.5.2 Hazards of cryogenic fluids

Cryogenic fluids should be kept in specially designed dewars, *not* domestic thermos flasks. Neither should fluids be kept enclosed without being vented to the atmosphere: one volume of liquid nitrogen boils off to give 700 volumes of gas, and is thus a potential explosive hazard. Furthermore, liquid nitrogen in large volumes can condense oxygen from the air, resulting in suffocation, and can cause cold burns in contact with skin. In severe cases the skin assumes a waxy appearance. Rewarming should be rapid, and medical advice sought immediately.

4.5.3 Orientation of tissue

Turner and Novacky (1973) describe a method (*Figure 4.10*) for orientating thin leaf sections that require rapid quenching to preserve labile cell structure. Strips of cellulose acetate paper 3 × 8 mm, impregnated with embedding medium, are placed on the vertical face of a brass rod 22 mm × 5 mm diameter. Excess medium is removed from the cellulose acetate papers with a squeegee. The specimen is sandwiched between them, and the second part of the rod sealed in place with adhesive tape bearing the sample number. The rods can be stored with their specimens in liquid nitrogen, or allowed to warm up for sectioning. The brass rod forms the chuck which is inserted into the cryostat, and the protruding cellulose acetate sandwich is set perpendicularly to the knife edge for cutting. The strip can either be cut as shown below, or reinforced with extra embedding media and trimmed to a mesa for cutting. Anken and Kappel (1993) recommend orientating specimens in gelatin capsules. The capsules are supported in 1 ml pipette tips (e.g. Eppendorf tips) stood in a polystyrene base. Once the specimen is orientated in the cooled embedding medium, it is snap-frozen and sectioned.

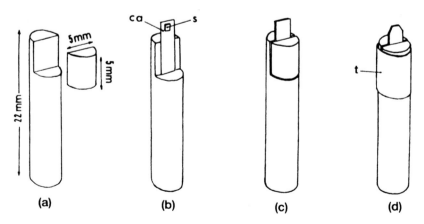

Figure 4.10: Freezing thin sections for cryotomy. (a) Components of the brass tissue carrier. (b) Cellulose acetate paper (ca) carries the sample (s) saturated with embedding compound. A second cellulose acetate paper strip is laid in place (c), and the entire carrier held in place with adhesive tape (t) for quenching (d). Reproduced from Turner and Novacky (1973) with permission from Williams & Wilkins.

4.6 Cryostat sectioning

Wedge knives, with or without a bevel, are used. The less the bevel, the better the anti-roll plate will lie on the surface of the knife. If the bevel is too great on the knife, then the rear part of the section may not be picked up when a slide is pressed onto the flat surface of the knife. A very finely stropped edge is useful for cold knife work, but will rapidly become blunt in the cryostat from frost and the frozen water of the hard tissue block. Disposable blades are useful where unfixed infectious specimens are to be cut, in which case two pairs of gloves should be worn, and the cryostat chamber disinfected with hot 10% formalin vapour after use. Because they are thin, and do not have the mass of the wedge immediately behind the cutting edge, disposable blades are not suitable for cutting very hard or fibrous tissue.

Trim the tissue on the chuck with a warm scalpel blade in a holder, taking care that the tissue does not thaw. Keep the supporting embedding medium to a minimum to reduce the possibility of sequential thick and thin sections. Where trimming is essential during sectioning, always reverse the block face before cutting again, or a very thick section will result.

Trimming should be done at not more than 10 µm. Thick trimming not only risks damaging and pitting the surface of the tissue, but the block may also become detached or loosened on the stub. Final facing of the tissue block should be done with the microtome advance set at 0 µm, then 1 µm, to remove any irregularities after trimming. Sequential areas of the blade are used to cut tissues, so making maximum use of the knife edge before resharpening or replacement.

As for paraffin wax sectioning, a very slow even stroke reduces compression and knife damage. At the cutting edge, the heat generated by the work required to fracture the tissue causes a zone of fusion. Tissues re-freeze further down the knife surface. A cold, clean knife and anti-roll plate is essential to produce good thin sections. After collection, a thin film of frost can be seen in the former position of the section. This should be brushed away with a good quality stiff brush about 1 cm wide. The knife should be brushed perpendicular and not parallel to the knife edge or else both will be ruined! It is possible to brush the wrinkles from sections 5–10 µm thick with a fine sable brush, before collecting with extreme care.

Condensation on the knife builds up if the knife is breathed upon when picking up sections, and will accrue normally, to a lesser extent, while sectioning. When cutting thin sections of less than 5 µm, or if the advance screw needs de-frosting, then thick and thin sections may result. Cryostat knives should be sharpened automatically, since a better straight edge is produced for the anti-roll plate to lie against.

4.6.1 Sectioning temperatures

Usually the higher the knife temperature, the colder the block must be. Fixed tissue cuts best at −10°C, since there is more water in fixed tissue, and the block is harder than fresh tissue at the same temperature. Most non-fatty fresh tissue cuts well at −18 to −25°C. Lipids must be cut at −25 to −30°C to give good sections, and very cold knife temperatures (less than −35°C) are required for cutting 1–2 μm sections and tissues of low freezing point from molluscs and fish. The relationship between section thickness and temperature which laid the basis for ultra-cryotomy, is not covered in this book. Interested readers should refer to Reid and Beesley (1991).

4.6.2 Anti-roll plate

A clean, well-maintained anti-roll plate is essential for good cryotomy (*Figure 4.11*). In the USA the anti-roll bar predominates, and serves the same purpose. The plate is made from Teflon-coated plastic or glass; the edges should be straight and free from nicks and scores, which can collect ice or impede the passage of the section. For this reason, some workers prefer to use disposable anti-roll plates rather than the custom design supplied with the cryostat (Schrader and Zeman, 1971). Whichever type of plate is used, the edges are covered in adhesive tape, which is 50 μm thick, sufficient to allow the section to pass between the knife and anti-roll plate surfaces. The edge of the plate should be set 0.5 mm below the edge of the knife, and the precise setting must be determined by trial and error. If the plate is set too high it will foul the face of the tissue block; if it is too low the section will curl up on the front edge of the anti-roll plate. The anti-roll bar is suited for larger tissue sections. As the section is cut, the bar lifts with the section onto the knife, preventing its loss from curling or scrambling due to electrostatic charge. The bar should be set about 1 mm below the edge of the knife, and particular attention paid to the tension of the bar as it rests on the section.

Usually, single sections are cut, but Zheng-yi (1993) has developed a modified anti-roll plate that permits ribbons of sections 3–4 μm thick from a paraffin block to be cut at −10°C in a cryostat. The degree of compression from a section cut using a cryostat compared to one cut at ambient temperature on a microtome is 8% and 50%, respectively.

4.6.3 Electrostatic charges

Where thin sections of about 3–5 μm are required or sections (particularly those with a high water content, or friable ones) are cut under dry atmospheric conditions, static can cause ruined sections, which scramble under the anti-roll plate. The causes of folded sections are thought to be the relatively low humidity, the friction generated between knife and block as the tissue is cut, and electrostatic attraction between the (negatively) charged anti-roll plate and positively charged ionic groups in the tissue.

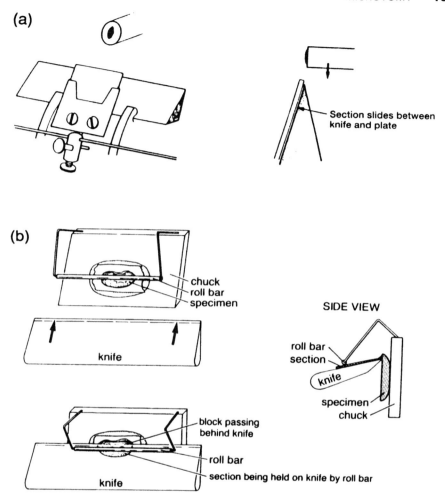

(a)

Section slides between
knife and plate

(b)

chuck
roll bar
specimen

knife

SIDE VIEW

roll bar
section

knife

specimen
chuck

block passing
behind knife

roll bar

section being held on knife by roll bar

knife

Figure 4.11:   The anti-roll plate (a) and anti-roll bar (b). Side views of the anti-roll plate and anti-roll bar in use, showing the methods of operation. Reproduced from (a) Culling *et al.* 1985 and (b) Watkins (1991) with permission from Butterworth-Heinemann Ltd and John Wiley & Sons, Inc. (Copyright © 1991 John Wiley & Sons, Inc.), respectively.

The cryostat chamber, knife, holder and anti-roll plate should all therefore be earthed. Static can be detected using a fibre of cotton wool attached to a metal microbial loop. It may be helpful to touch the anti-roll plate prior to collecting each section. Cleaning the knife surface and the anti-roll plate with cold acetone at −20°C prior to cutting can also help reduce static. Viebahn and Lüttenberg (1989) recommend coating the anti-roll plate with a 100 nm transparent layer of gold-chromium, or a commercially deposited layer of metal oxide. The former metal layer tends to wear off, and must be deposited on home-made glass plates made from microscope slides.

Table 4.1: Different methods of collecting and handling frozen sections after sectioning

(i)	Pick up section on warm or cold slide or coverslip. Thaw and dry in air
(ii)	Pick up section on warm or cold slide or coverslip, thaw, dry in air and post-fix
(iii)	Pick up section on warm or cold slide or coverslip. Fix by immersion at the moment of thawing
(iv)	Pick up section on warm or cold slide or coverslip. Immerse in cold protective medium. Fix and process later
(v)	Pick up on materials other than glass (e.g. cellulose acetate film, stripping film, semi-permeable membrane)
(vi)	Deliver directly, or transfer on a slide (or other support) into warm or cold incubating medium, or buffer, for enzyme histochemistry
(vii)	Deliver directly, or transfer into warm or cold fixative
(viii)	Deliver directly, or transfer into warm or cold immunocytochemical reagent or stain
(ix)	Freeze dry or freeze substitute
(x)	Microwave

Adapted from Pearse (1980) with permission from Churchill Livingstone.

4.6.4 Handling sections

The different methods discussed below are listed in *Table 4.1*. The most common way to collect frozen sections is to mount them directly onto a 'warm' slide (at room temperature) positioned directly over the section and pressed onto the surface of the knife. The section will be seen to 'jump' onto the slide as it thaws directly upon contact. The best-cut thin sections (a few micrometers) will take a fraction of a second, while thicker ones (greater than 10 μm) will take a second or so to thaw. The sections are then air-dried and post-fixed as appropriate. Sections may also be picked up into chilled or warm buffer or fixative. This technique is usually applied to thick sections cut in gelatin, and not the commercial PEG embedding media which are soluble in aqueous fluids. Sections that are embedded in the latter types of medium are liable to suffer from stretching artifacts once they are held in a free-floating state before mounting.

Another aid to collecting sections has been published by Fink (1992), using an aqueous coating spray and an organic pressure-sensitive adhesive to mount cryo-sections onto slides without thawing before further treatment. It is also possible to freeze dry and freeze substitute sections after cutting—with good preservation of morphology and structural relationships of labile cell constituents. These latter techniques are advanced methods; the reader is referred to Pearse (1980) and Bancroft (1990) for comprehensive reviews. Microwaving of cryostat sections is dealt with in Section 2.14, but requires rapid and dexterous manipulation.

4.6.5 Storage of tissue

Tissues held for more than a few hours in the cryostat will dry out, and gelatin or agar blocks will shrink. The protocol given in Section 3.13 will serve for storing gelatin blocks in the refrigerator. Tissues should be stored embedded or otherwise in airtight plastic screwtop vials (Nunc®), or in heat-sealed polythene tubing at −80°C in a cold cabinet, or at −196°C

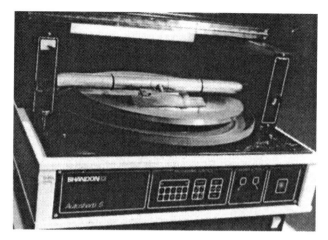

Figure 4.12:   The Shandon automatic knife sharpener (photograph courtesy of Dr Savile Bradbury).

immersed in liquid nitrogen. A layer of physiological saline is poured onto the frozen block, and the whole is snap-frozen again. The container can then be stored at –20°C without damage.

4.7 Knife sharpening

Knives have to be kept as sharp as possible in order to cut good quality sections. The advantage of a small cutting angle is lost with a blunt knife, and the effects of compression and distortion are increased. Automatic sharpening machines (*Figure 4.12*) give the best and most consistent results, but it is possible to sharpen knives by hand.

Hand sharpening is very time-consuming, and requires extensive experience. Brief details are given here, but more complete accounts may be found in Clayden (1971) and Gray (1972). Sharpening consists of two independent operations: honing and stropping. Honing involves moving the knife over a hard surface with abrasive to remove sufficient metal to replace the rounded cutting edge. Stropping involves polishing the re-made edge, with or without abrasive, on a softer surface to give a crisp cutting edge. Often it is sufficient merely to strop the knife before cutting. Beginners are advised to sharpen their knives on a good automatic machine, and to strop the edge carefully before use. Sharpening should then rarely be required, unless the bevel is much reduced or the edge ruined, or turned by poor stropping (see *Figure 4.14*). New knives will require sharpening to improve the factory edge; they should be sharpened on a completely flat glass plate lapped by diamond bar or plate (Section 4.7.5).

Honing should only be required when the section quality is diminished and the knife no longer feels sharp. The macroscopic appearance of the section should be sufficient to indicate when honing is required. Nicks in the knife will cause scores or tearing of soft, dense tissue such as spleen; increased compression, distortion and difficulty in ribboning will also be evident. A dull edge will often re-orientate connective tissue fibres in the direction of the knife, and this can be seen in lymph node and spleen.

Before sharpening, the knife should be cleaned with xylene to remove surplus wax, washed and thoroughly dried. Inspect the knife with a hand lens or inverted eyepiece and mark any nicks with an indelible pen. Some workers recommend using a platform to support the knife while viewing it under a stereo microscope; this is not a good idea, as the knife edge can easily suffer or cause damage.

Half-inch plate glass is a suitable support surface for sharpening knives. Automatic machines use a large flat circular cast-iron plate impregnated with carborundum grit. The advantage of glass or cast-iron plates over the classical carborundum stone is threefold.

1. The surface area of a carborundum stone is insufficient to allow the whole of the knife edge to be sharpened at once.
2. Large, accurately flat stones are expensive, and are easily worn away from a truly flat surface.
3. Abrasive properties are limited.

Metal plates quickly retain the powders used for sharpening, but a new glass surface must be matted with a fine abrasive powder until it is just rough enough to retain the abrasive powders. If the surface is too rough, or is worn with use, then the powder may not come into contact with the knife facet. In this case the plate should be lapped with another glass surface until it becomes less rough. Conversely, if the surface of the plate is too smooth, the abrasive will not be held sufficiently in place to cut the knife surface properly.

4.7.1 Lubricants

The functions of the lubricants used during sharpening are to keep the knife edge cool (and so avoid loss of temper), to assist the flow of particles away from the knife edge, and to prevent the stone or plate from becoming blocked and thus ensure a smooth, sharpening action. Commercial lubricants should be non-aqueous, since aqueous lubricants will not only promote rust, but may affect the surface of the plate. A soluble or thin lubricating oil can be used. The abrasive should ideally be applied as a single layer, with sufficient space to allow lubricant to flow freely.

Too much powder leads to inefficient abrasion. If much metal has to be removed from the knife, it pays to change the abrasive often, as the largest particles perform the most work. However, these large particles soon become small and spherical, reducing the speed of abrasion. This is what is required to produce a smooth facet, so ultimately the requirements change. Once a sufficient bevel has been ground onto the knife, prolonged abrasion with finer and finer particles is required to produce a well-polished facet.

Water should always be double-distilled and filtered to remove particles; it should not be used on metal plates. A 15% solution of Teepol (sodium alkyl sulphate), or 50% glycerin in water is useful for glass plates only, but should not be used on metal or stone. Thin neutral oils, such as a light machine oil, are suited to metal plates or stones. The commercial mixture 'Hyprez' is suitable for both metal and glass plates. Further mixtures are given in Gray (1972).

4.7.2 Types of abrasive

Diamond dust supplied either as coloured paste or aerosols is the most expensive and the best abrasive available. Particles from 50 to 0.25 μm are used; the cutting action can be maintained for hours, and the particles are far less prone than other types to break down and become rounded. Diamond paste can be purchased in colour-coded syringe applicators to reduce waste in use. Carborundum is recommended only for initial grinding, as the large particles break down readily; sizes range from 20 (2 F) to 7 (4 F) μm. Various metal oxides can also be used; the particle sizes range from 0.3 to 0.05 μm, and are excellent for final polishing. White Bauxilite, or aluminium oxide, is available in a coarse 850 or fine 1200 grade, and Durmax alumina, a better quality oxide, is supplied in liquid form to be used on Kemet or glass plates. There are four grades from coarse (6 μm) to extra fine (0.5 μm).

The amount of powder used should be very small, and resemble a thin paste. If too much abrasive is used, the powder will not cut deeply enough into the knife; if too little is used, the cuts will be deep, but insufficient to give a good edge. Whenever changing from one type of abrasive powder to another, the plate must be thoroughly cleaned to avoid cross-contamination. Both the plate and knife must be wiped with lubricant. If it is possible to wash, rinse and thoroughly dry the plate and knife, then detergent and water can be used to clean the plate and knife betwen changing abrasive powders.

4.7.3 Handles and backs

The purpose of the knife back is to lift the knife away from the sharpening surface to produce the correct facet. Each knife should have its own back so that it lies perfectly on the sharpening plane, and the minimum of metal is removed to produce a perfect facet. Where the facets are asymmetrical, which is rare, the back can be fitted only one way. In any case, for both types of facet, there is usually a reference mark on the knife back to ensure that it is fitted onto the knife in a particular way. This is because no knife is completely straight and true; the knife edge and back should therefore wear at an equal rate and in the same way.

During sharpening, both facets must be sharpened alternately to prevent an excessive burr forming on the reverse edge. Tool edge and plano-concave knives are only sharpened on one edge, and so the burr must be removed by careful light honing. Deeply biconcave Heiffor knives (profile BL) are rarely used now; they do not require a back to sharpen them, but do require more practice to keep the facet held at a constant angle during sharpening. The handle of a Heiffor knife is either integral, or screws into the blade for sharpening. The manufacturers of 'D' profile knives recommend hand sharpening, but designs of suitable knife-backs (Pearse, 1973) for automatic sharpening have been published.

4.7.4 Manual sharpening

A piece of plate glass or a stone $40 \times 15 \times 1$ cm is anchored on the bench top, or placed on a damp cloth to prevent it slipping, and the surface charged with an abrasive and lubricant mixed to a fine suspension with the fingertips. Carborundum, Arkansas or Belgian Black Vein stones are available; the latter are the best: they are yellow and contain ferric oxide.

The hone should be wiped over with xylene before use to remove any particles or dust. The speed of honing or stropping is not crucial; however, excessive pressure should not be used to hold the knife to the glass or stone, but just sufficient to make the hone bite the edge of the knife. Push the knife away on the knife edge with the back trailing, turn it over and draw it towards you at an angle (*Figure 4.13*). If the hone is too small, not only will it wear away in the centre, but the knife will show a curved facet and

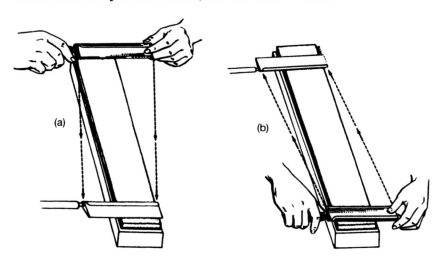

Figure 4.13: Manual knife honing. The knife is held (with forefinger and thumb, to facilitate easy rotation) flat onto the hone under its own weight and pushed with a light pressure and regular movement, with the back of the knife trailing (a). At the end of the stone, the knife is turned over on its back, flat against the stone as before, and drawn towards the operator (b). The sequence is repeated as often as necessary. Reproduced from Luna (1968) *Manual of Histologic Staining Methods of the Armed Forces Institute of Pathology,* 3rd edn, McGraw-Hill, New York; with permission from Mosby-Year Book, Inc.

edge. The hone should be at least as wide as the long edge of the knife. A narrow hone is disadvantageous for several reasons: there is a danger of tipping the knife on the edge of the stone; the final facet may be curved since the centre of the stone wears faster; and the facet may be wider in the centre due to the constant wear here compared to the outer part of the knife. Cover the honing stone when it is not in use.

Final polishing should be done with Linde Alpha (0.3 µm) and Gamma (0.05 µm) on a glass plate, or with fine diamond abrasive on a very fine (Arkansas) stone. The microscopic appearance of the knife after initial honing should present a matt 1 mm facet with a scratch-free cutting edge, and a uniform pattern of serrations, without protrusions. The final facet should reflect a high polish without nicks or serrations.

4.7.5 Lapping

A stone or plate will eventually require lapping, as a central depression is ground into the surface, which can transfer to the knife. A stone can be lapped by rubbing alternately between two other stones (rubbing two stones alone will cause one to assume a concave and the other a convex surface). If the knife edge is very slightly curved it can be remedied with care by drawing it across the long axis of the sharpening stone, and re-honing.

The plates of sharpening machines are lapped true with a lapping plate or bar. The bar is impregnated with diamond, and should be used with a coarse abrasive at maximum pressure, followed by using the reverse side and a fine abrasive. The lapping bar tends not to remove the surface depression in a glass plate. Banthorpe and Court (1970) recommend using a sheet of plate glass 40 × 10 cm with a 2 F coarse aluminium oxide paste, worked by hand over the plate, to remove the shine of the centrally worn surface. Shandon have produced a lapping plate called the 'Microsharp' Kemet plate which is an aluminium disc impregnated with copper parti- cles. The plate is charged with 3 µm diamond paste and a lubricant. Since the particles do not rotate under the edge of the knife, they produce far less scoring than ordinary abrasion, and can be used where a knife needs only a small amount of honing.

4.7.6 Stropping

Some people object to stropping, or polishing, the edge; indeed, after good honing it may not be necessary. Certainly, if a knife is badly stropped then the preceding honing is rendered worthless, for the edge will be turned (*Figure 4.14*) and blunted as before, and the clearance angle will be impossible to set (see *Figure 4.16*). The strop can be supported on a hook (the hanging type), or on a slide or wooden back (*Figure 4.15*). The hanging strop may have two leather sides: dress one side with a fine, and the other

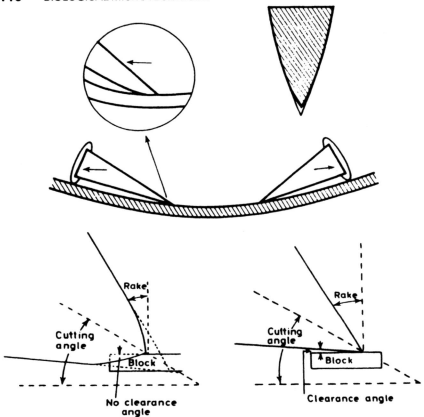

Figure 4.14: The effects of poor stropping. If the knife is not held flat, or the strop kept taught, or the knife is held with too much pressure, the edge will become rounded (top). This will prevent the proper clearance angle from being set (bottom). The knife edge is a minute circle with a circumference of about 0.2 μm arc. The arc of a rounded, blunt edge may approach the thickness of a section (Gray, 1972).

with an extra fine paste. Otherwise, the strop is constructed with coarse linen and fine leather sides. Where the hanging type is used, ensure that the fixing will allow it to be pulled taught without giving, and that it is used in an area away from doors and passages.

All strops should be covered when not in use to keep them free from dust or dirt, which would otherwise ruin the knife edge. A strop should be dressed with a small quantity of paste, since a dry strop can ruin the edge. Do not use mineral oil, and use only a very fine paste. The strop should either have two leather sides made of horse hide (horse-shell), or have one side of canvas. The canvas (or coarse-dressed) side should be used first. Cork can also be used on a rigid base.

Fit the knife back to maintain the correct facet angle, and use the strop taut with the knife back leading, and the edge trailing, to prevent the knife cutting into the strop. The knife should be moved across the strop at a very

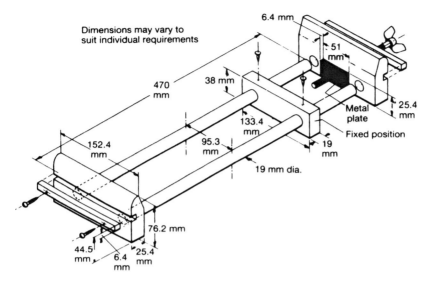

Figure 4.15: Design of a strop holder. Reproduced from Luna (1968) *Manual of Histologic Staining Methods of the Armed Forces Institute of Pathology*, 3rd edn, McGraw-Hill, New York; with permission from Mosby-Year Book, Inc.

slight angle (*Figure 4.16*). After stropping, the knife should be washed by directing a stream of water over its back edge to the front. Dry the bulk of the knife on a lint-free cloth, avoiding the edge, and follow with an acetone wash to dry the edge. Many people advocate cutting a free hair or feeling the edge of a knife; the only true test is the quality of section as it is cut, and the degree of compression that results.

4.8 Sectioning

The most common section thickness for wax sections is 3–8 μm and resin sections from 0.5 to 3 μm; unfixed frozen sections may be cut from 3 to 12 μm, and fixed frozen sections from 10 to 50 μm. These figures are only a guide, but in general, hard dense matrices can be cut more thinly than soft blocks. The density of the embedding medium should ideally match that of the tissue so that compression is minimized, and tissue is not torn out of a soft supporting medium.

Most paraffin wax mixtures used for sectioning have melting points in the range of 45–60°C. In a temperate climate, a wax mixture which melts at 55–56°C is used. Harder waxes are easier to cut, but involve higher temperatures during embedding. Sectioning of the gut of experimental animals is made easier if they are starved or fed soft, cooked food free of cellulose or lignin at least 24 h before killing.

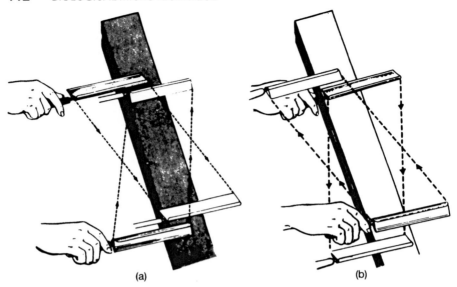

(a)   (b)

Figure 4.16: Stropping a knife. The strop (here shown on a second type of support) should be with the cutting edge of the knife trailing (a), and in a diagonal movement to sharpen the entire length of the edge (b). The operation is thus a reversal of honing; generally 8–12 times in each direction is sufficient. Reproduced from Luna (1968) *Manual of Histologic Staining Methods of the Armed Forces Institute of Pathology*, 3rd edn, McGraw-Hill, New York; with permission from Mosby-Year Book, Inc.

There are six physical factors concerning the knife which determine the efficiency with which it may be used to section blocks, and which are independent of the manner in which the block has been processed. These are as follows.

(i)   Cutting (wedge or bevel) angle.
(ii) Sharpness and temper.
(iii) Facet polish and coating (if any).
(iv) Clearance angle.
(v)   Rake angle.
(vi) Knife obliquity (slope angle = effective cutting angle for a sliding microtome).

4.8.1 Wax structure

Wax for histology is derived from one of the last hydrocarbon fractions of the refinement of crude oil (Allison, 1978). The waxes are sold with melting points from 40 to 70°C; the melting point of a particular wax is determined by the hydrocarbon content and nature of additives and plasticizers blended into the mixture.

The cutting quality of a particular wax is determined not only by its melting point, but also its microcrystalline structure. Severe compression of sections occurs in pure paraffin wax, which is highly crystalline; compression also occurs, by up to 15%, when the hot wax used for embedding cools. Ideally, a small crystal structure is required, but not so small that cohesive strength between crystals in the wax is lost. Too high an embedding temperature can lead to the tissue becoming brittle, and the wax becoming over-oxidized so that it no longer hardens adequately.

Various additives have been added to paraffin wax. A historical review and list of protocols for wax mixtures has been published by Lamb (1973). Nowadays, synthetic resins are used as plasticizers. These additives lodge between crystals to prevent their full growth, and plasticizers provide better adhesion of the wax mass. Dempster concluded (Allison, 1979) that the transition point is of greater relevance to sectioning properties than the melting point. Above the transition temperature, cutting is by shearing along the cleavage plane in a point-to-point fashion, whereas below this temperature, cutting is by discontinuous fracturing. Decreasing the knife bevel, and using a sharp knife and a polished front facet will decrease the amount of shear, and hence serve to reduce compression.

The wax at the surface of the block is composed of concentric, laminated, ordered structures, while the upper matt surface of a wax section displays an ordered, yet irregular, crystalline structure which is absent from the shiny lower surface. Heating effects from cutting the section raise the temperature above the transition point and cause slip readjustment between crystals at the lower surface. This is the cause of non-recoverable compression. Where shear and prismatic slip act on a thick section, excessive curling may take place (in a manner akin to chiselling) as shear forces become excessive. The degree of compression is also due to the magnitude of bending that the section undergoes as it is cleaved from the block. This is related not only to the rake angle, but also the evenness and speed of the cutting stroke.

Unless the wax is held at a temperature between that of its melting and plastic transition points, it will become whitish opaque when struck suddenly (as in microtomy). This opacity is due to the formation of minute cleavages and air spaces at intercrystalline junctions and lamellae. These cleavages are more pronounced, and further slip occurs with a decrease in the rake angle. Curling is increased above 8 µm, especially with hard or decalcified tissues and those embedded in cellulose or resin. Lowering the cutting and ambient temperature has a similar effect to increasing the rake angle, which should be as large as possible. A blunt knife has the effect of grossly reducing the rake angle which serves to promote prismatic break-up of the sections. The increased slip and shear cause sections to be cut much thicker than the nominal setting on the microtome, and distortion, as well as compression, of the sections is increased.

4.8.2 Compression

Most blocks are cut across their short axis, but this may sometimes need to be altered to the long axis (e.g. a needle biopsy) where compression

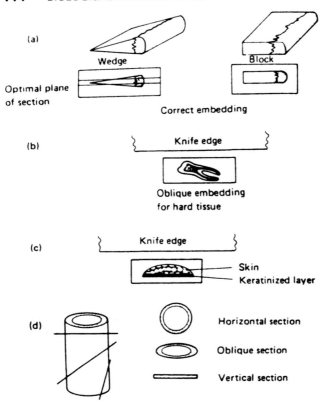

Figure 4.17: Orientation of heterogenous tissue. Skin and mucosa should be orientated (a) to display the constituent layers in transverse section. Straight-edged samples are preferable to wedges for microtomy. Hard tissues (e.g. bone, uterus, wood) are best orientated obliquely (b) to reduce or prevent 'chattering' and possible damage to the knife. Tissues (e.g. skin), which have combined hard and soft constiuents, should be orientated as in (c), so that tearing of the softer tissues is prevented. Tubes should be sectioned transversely (d) to display the lumen clearly. Reproduced from Culling *et al.* (1985) with permission from Butterworth-Heinemann Ltd.

across the short axis results in an uninterpretable section. Heterogenous tissues, containing hard and soft components (e.g. keratinized skin, epithelium and dermis in a skin biopsy) will need to be cut at 45° to the tissue layers so that the section does not tear (*Figure 4.17*).

The effect of block orientation upon the degree of compression is important. When a rectangular block is orientated to be cut through the short axis, then compression is in the short axis alone. When cut through the long axis, compression occurs in the long axis with re-distribution in the short axis, which is increased. However, sectioning through the corner may damage the contours and relationships of many components, particularly with inhomogenous tissues. Therefore, unless particularly tough tissue components necessitate a particular orientation (e.g. skin), sectioning is either carried out through the short axis, or through the corner. It is preferable to block out specimens such that the tissue is presented at a slant to the block faces, rather than slant the knife (where this is possible) so that ribboning will occur.

The shearing action of the knife of a sliding microtome, set at an angle to reduce the effective cutting angle, is well known and has been studied by Dempster (1942b). Not only does compression occur along the longitudinal cutting axis, but lateral re-orientation also occurs depending upon the obliquity of the knife, both being greatest for a knife set at 45°, and thin sections. The best set is to use the knife at an angle of about 20° from the transverse plane.

There is always a degree of permanent compression introduced into a section due to the manner in which the embedding matrix is cleaved from the block. A blunt blade and a grossly excessive rake angle (> 30°) will cause the knife to 'chisel out', rather than cleave, the section from the block. Due to the friction exerted by the blade, the thickness of the section (and hence internal resilience of the section to frictional drag) will determine how much a section will compress. The usual amount of compression seen in paraffin wax sections, sectioned at ambient temperature is as follows.

12–25 µm	15–20%
5 µm	60%
2.5 µm	84%
(5 µm cut at −10°C for comparison	8–10%)

These values hold good whether a sledge or rotary microtome is used, with sections under 10 µm being more variable. Very thin sections compress so much more because of the effect of local warming. A cold knife will dissipate heat generated by friction, and so will further reduce compression, as will a reduced rake.

Although reduced knife bevels are an advantage, if they are too low, and the cutting speed too high, the knife will spring as it meets and overcomes resistance in the block. Moreover, too small a knife bevel will increase the radius of curvature (Dempster, 1942a). This results in the formation of slight transverse grooves between the slip planes formed by prismatic slip formation. The composition of the wax is important, too; soft waxes cleave in a point-to-point fashion, and the ambient temperature has a greater effect on the cutting qualities of soft than hard mixtures. Harder mixtures are therefore better for cutting thin sections, and the degree of compression for ice-chilled blocks is correspondingly about 10–15% less than those cut at room temperature (Merriam, 1957).

Deformation from the shearing effect of the microtome blade on the tissue was reported at about 6% by Ross (1953), whereas Boonstra et al. (1983) found a decrease of up to 4%, in the cutting direction, with cervical tissue. Shape deformation is enhanced when cutting thin sections embedded in a high-melting point (hard) wax, and when the sections are overheated during mounting; in this case they are liable to expand then contract excessively on cooling. Smith (1962) recommended that tissues should be dried at room temperature at a moderately high humidity to reduce both shrinkage and variability in staining. Collins (1969) reported that if the blade is etched, compression is reduced by a factor of 3–5 from typical compression values of 10–25% to 2–8%.

Glass 'Ralph' knives also cause less compression than steel knives; the compression quotients of paraffin and resin sections using glass knives have been quoted as 6–28% and 4–19%, respectively (Helander, 1984). This range was due to the cutting angle formed on a series of knives, and hence a series of knives can be broken to suit different tissues.

Flattening out on a water bath (Section 3.8) is carried out at about 10°C below the melting temperature of the wax; since this is above the plastic transition temperature, the section can stretch as the tissue absorbs water and expands. Where the paraffin is much softer than the embedded tissue, the latter will be compressed and show corrugations—these can be partly recovered if the surrounding matrix is teased away on the water bath.

4.8.3 Clearance angle

Since the bevel angle of the knife is set, the clearance (tilt) and rake angle are the only ones that can be altered by the microtomist. For knives with bevel angles of about 30°, the best clearance angle is usually about 4°, although it is possible to reduce this to about 1° if care is taken that wax accretions do not accumulate on the rear face of the knife. The beginner may wish to use *Figure 4.18* for setting the clearance angle.

4.8.4 Sectioning technique

Paraffin wax.
1. Ensure that the embedded blocks are chilled or soaked as required. Avoid excess soaking, which will produce tissue blocks with a soggy surface.
2. Insert the knife into its holder, and check that the clearance, rake and slant angle are correctly set. Ensure that the feed screw is wound back fully.
3. Trim off excess wax from around the specimen, and square up the block face as described in Section 3.6. Fix the block in the holder securely.
4. Move the block holder forwards or upwards until it nearly touches the knife. Ensure that the block face moves parallel to the edge of the knife, and that the top edge is parallel to ensure ribboning. Do not dig the blade into the face of the block!
5. Trim the face of the block, with one reserved part of the knife, in steps of 10–15 µm until sufficient tissue is exposed. Some workers use a separate knife for this, which is permissible if a lot of blocks are being trimmed at once, but to do so involves re-setting the knife, and losing some tissue, which may be precious. Do not trim too coarsely, the block may be torn, tissue completely lost and/or the knife damaged. Nick one

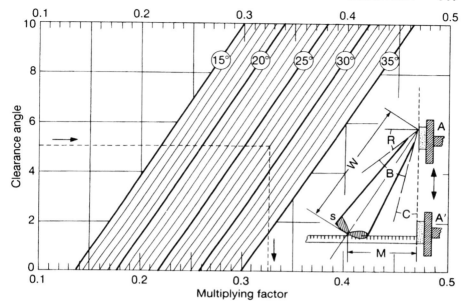

Figure 4.18: Setting the clearance angle. For the desired clearance angle (e.g. 5°) follow the abscissa to the oblique line giving the bevel or wedge angle (B) of the knife. Read down to the multiplying factor (i.e. 0.327). This factor multiplied by the width (W) of the knife will give the distance (M) in millimetres to be set between the midpoint of the heel and perpendicular to the block face. R, rake angle; C, clearance angle; S, notches in the heel of the knife to assist setting the knife whilst moving the block between A and A', the limits of the cutting stroke. Reproduced from Dempster (1942a) with permission from Wiley-Liss, a division of John Wiley and Sons, Inc. Copyright © 1942 Wiley-Liss.

corner of the block so that sections may be teased apart on the water-bath and orientated correctly on the slide.

6. The block should then be re-chilled, and the next block, if any, trimmed.

7. Reset the thickness gauge to 0 or 1 μm, check the tightness and security of block, holder and knife, and 'polish' the face of the block before taking routine sections at 4–5 μm. A regular rhythm is required; any jerky motion will cause thick and thin sectioning, gouges or missed sections—resulting in an extra thick part of a section next time around.

8. Just before the section comes off, 'huff' on the block and lift off the section with a fine brush. This causes a more even density in the surface of the block, and aids sectioning. Once the wax is ribboning, support it with a brush or seeker. Take four to five sections for floating out, and tease the best ones apart with a pair of forceps and seeker.

9. Due to different knife tempers, some knives will cut soft tissue better than tough, and vice versa. Keep a note of which knives are best suited for which purposes.

Thin sections from 1 to 3 µm tend to curl, and need more care in lifting off the knife with a paintbrush and supporting with a seeker before they will ribbon. Residual moisture from blocks chilled on ice will cause sections to stick to the knife, and it is best to chill either in a refrigerator or on a Petri dish cooled on ice. If a wooden chuck is used, soak it in hot wax under vacuum to impregnate with wax and remove the water.

Cellulose sections.
1. Keep the block, knife and sections wet throughout with a fine camel-hair brush dipped in 70% alcohol, between taking each section.
2. Fix the block into the block holder, and ensure the knife is set at a 30–40° slant, with a slight clearance angle.
3. Turn back the feed mechanism as far as possible and move the block face up to the knife edge and set parallel with it. Check and tighten all adjustments as required.
4. Set the thickness gauge to 15 µm, flood the knife and block with 70% alcohol, and face off the tissue.
5. Cut the sections at 12–15 µm slowly and smoothly, and hold the sections down with a brush as they come off the knife; otherwise they will curl.
6. Brush the sections from the knife into 70% alcohol. Store them either in individual trays, or adhered to squares of 'hard' toilet paper numbered with Indian ink. These can then be stacked up in a single container.

Serial cellulose sections can be collected, in order, to one side of the knife on translucent paper (Feeney, 1944) and mounted by inversion onto the slide. The speed of cutting should ideally be as slow as is possible consistent with a smooth action, as stopping will cause chattering and gouges. Harder tissue may benefit from slightly faster cutting. The cutting speed is also influenced by block consistency, ambient temperature and humidity. Polyester, ester wax and PEG should be cut at half-speed, and with a cooled knife, preferably at a temperature less than 22°C. Microtomes should be cleaned completely of wax at the finish of each cutting session. Brush off the majority of the wax with a brush kept for the purpose. Oil the slides and moving parts lightly with machine oil, and cover the instrument when finished.

Resin sections.
The sections are usually collected dry using a very slow, but consistent, sectioning speed, although they may be cut into a trough of water. As the dry section comes away from the knife it should be lifted clear, with either a fine brush or watchmaker's forceps, to reduce the formation of wrinkles. Some authors contend that dry sectioning results in inconsistent section thickness and problems with static, and use 40% ethanol to moisten the knife and collect the sections as they are cut. The blocks are trimmed with a slanting top edge so that they do not catch on the knife edge as they are transferred off the blade.

Sectioning is best performed on a heavy motorized retractable micro-tome to ensure reproducible sections of accurate thickness. A glass knife on a retracting microtome should be used for sections from 0.5 to 2 μm; sections up to 3 μm can be cut on a disposable steel blade, and those that are thicker still on a D-profile steel blade. Depending upon the conditions, the speed will vary from 2 to 20 mm sec^{-1}. The recommended clearance angle is 4–7° for 45° glass, and 10–15° for 30° steel knives, which are greater than the values given for cutting paraffin sections. Resin sections should be cut at 2–5 mm sec^{-1} using glass, and 0.5–2 mm sec^{-1} with diamond knives. With a glass knife the optimal PEG plasticizer concentration is 4% and for steel knives is increased to 7% to produce a slightly softer block.

Since semi-thin sections do not form ribbons, they have to be collected in sequential order in a tray with a series of wells. These trays can be made in one of two ways: fine holes can be punctured in the bottom of a multiwell serological plate with a needle, or else a fine nylon mesh can be solvent-welded onto a shallow cylindrical perspex body. The sections are then lifted into the trays of water or 50% ethanol with a 'hockey stick', a Pasteur pipette whose end has been melted into a small ball, a wire loop, an eyelash mounted in a cocktail stick or a stainless steel spatula with holes drilled into it. Care has to be taken that the sections do not fold into a knot as they are floated out, and some workers fling the resin section onto the water surface.

4.9 Section thickness

It is commonly assumed that the desired section thickness, which is selected when cutting, is reproducible without significant variance. In fact this is not so, even when the knife is freshly sharpened. It is particularly important for quantitative work to know the extent to which section thickness changes from the nominal value set on the microtome. The easiest way to measure section thickness is either by focusing on the upper and lower section planes, or by turning the cut edge of a section through 90° and measuring this. The former method has an inherent error of at least 10%, and is described in detail by Lange and Engström (1954). The latter technique is described by Merriam (1957), who found that adjacent sections at the same microtome setting can have different thicknesses, and that variations within a section also occur; this intra-section variation increases with an increase in the thickness of cut, and is as much as ± 3 μm for a 30 μm section (10%) to 0.5 μm for a 1 μm section (50%).

Studies on paraffin and GMA (Helander, 1983), and frozen sections (Pearse and Marks, 1974; Antony *et al.*, 1984) have investigated the variations found in section thickness. The actual departure in the thickness of paraffin sections from the nominal setting of 5 μm ranged from 3 to 7 μm, with a mean of 4.8 μm and standard error of 0.14 μm. In paraffin sections, half the cell nucleii may be partly torn from the section or left intact, giving rise to surface variations. This variation is of the order of 1–2 μm with a fresh disposable blade, well-sharpened steel knife or glass 'Ralph' knife. With a used steel blade, or one that has not been stropped, the variation in thickness can exceed 3 μm. The structure of a plastic block is much more amorphous than any paraffin wax mixture, and work by Helander (1983) showed that thickness and surface variations were both less than 0.3 μm. The results of Helander's study on paraffin sections is similar to that of Merriam (1957) who earlier showed a range of 4–9 μm, with a mean of 7.0 μm and SEM of 0.16 μm for a microtome setting of 5 μm.

4.9.1 Cryostat sectioning

Differences in the actual thickness of cryostat sections also occur. There is a tendency for the greatest discrepancy to occur in those tissues, such as skin, which are heterogeneous having connective tissue in close proximity to dense cellular tissue. Other tissues, such as lymphoid tissue, may either cut very thick or thin. Pearse and Marks (1974) showed that tissues tended to be approximately 30% thinner than indicated on the instrument due to water loss on drying, and that this difference was largely consistent between different tissues, with a greater variation for skin. Anthony et al. (1984) quoted a greater reduction in section thickness down to 10%, with inter/intra-section variability as 11% and 7% for a rocker and 5% and 4% for a rotary microtome, respectively. In my experience, unless the knife is well stropped and very new, sections are often much thicker than the nominal setting; the easiest practical way to determine this is by observing the rate at which the section thaws onto the slide. A very thick section will not only curl ominously when cut, but will also take a couple of seconds to thaw onto the slide. The cutting speed of the microtome, as well as knife quality, has a bearing not only on compression, but section thickness. The faster the cutting speed, the thicker the section. Butcher (1971) has shown that section thickness can depart by up to 5 μm from the nominal setting, depending upon the cutting speed used.

4.10 Effect of fixation and processing on tissue size

Most of the tissue shrinkage that is the unavoidable side-effect of specimen preparation results from embedding in hot wax. The shrinkage due to fixation is about 3–5%, despite the formaldehyde being 1300 mOsm, and often up to 2000–3000 mOsm, compared with the range of 250–350 mOsm for tissues.

Not all components of tissue swell or shrink equally, leaving artifactual spaces. Dehydration and paraffin embedding will always produce some shrinkage of tissue; the exact amount is determined by the type of tissue and the processing schedule. In general, fixatives swell tissues, and tissue stored for any length of time in fixative must be put in a container with a wide enough neck to allow for at least a 50% increase in volume.

Ross (1953) measured both linear and volumetric changes, and found that Sanfelice's fluid caused appreciably less shrinkage of cell and nuclear diameter of loosely organized tissue than other cytological fixatives, with the nucleus shrinking less than the cytoplasm (*Table 4.2*). Ross concluded that the role of the fixative is subordinate to the subsequent processing, but that cells processed into paraffin wax shrank more after being fixed with simple fixatives than with balanced fixative mixtures. Linear shrinkage of whole cells after paraffin processing was about 25–45%; volume shrinkage was 61–78%.

Approximate figures have been given for linear tissue shrinkage at each stage of processing *after fixation* by Iwadare *et al.* (1984), for kidney and liver, which are both dense tissues (*Figure 4.19*). They found that at the final paraffin embedding the tissues had shrunk consistently by 12–16% whatever schedule was used. About 1–2% shrinkage occurs during dehy-

Table 4.2: Shrinkage of primary spermatocytes of *Helix aspersa* after different fixation conditions

	Whole cells		Nuclei	
Fixative	% shrinkage diameter	% shrinkage volume	% shrinkage diameter	% shrinkage volume
Acetic acid	34 ± 4	71 ± 5	23 ± 7	54 ± 12
Bouin's	27 ± 9	61 ± 14	23 ± 7	54 ± 12
Chromic acid	34 ± 4	71 ± 5	23 ± 7	54 ± 12
Ethanol	40 ± 6	78 ± 6	34 ± 6	71 ± 8
Helly's	27 ± 9	61 ± 14	28 ± 9	63 ± 14
Mercuric-acetic	27 ± 9	61 ± 14	28 ± 9	63 ± 14
Mercuric chloride	34 ± 4	71 ± 5	28 ± 9	63 ± 14
Mercuric-formol	22 ± 4	53 ± 7	23 ± 7	54 ± 12
Neutral formalin	30 ± 4	66 ± 6	23 ± 7	54 ± 12
Osmium tetroxide	27 ± 9	61 ± 14	28 ± 9	63 ± 14
Picric acid	40 ± 6	78 ± 6	34 ± 6	71 ± 8
Potassium dichromate	40 ± 6	78 ± 6	31 ± 9	67 ± 13
Sanfelice's	13 ± 5	34 ± 11	9 ± 3	25 ± 7
Trichloroacetic acid	34 ± 4	71 ± 5	34 ± 6	71 ± 8
Zenker's	27 ± 9	61 ± 14	23 ± 7	54 ± 12

Cells embedded in paraffin wax tend to shrink more after fixation in simple (primary) fixatives than when fixed in fixative mixtures. In keeping with other studies, cytoplasmic shrinkage is generally greater than that of the nucleus. There is no significant difference in shrinkage between cells following immersion in most fixatives. The linear shrinkage of the entire cell is generally by one-third.
Data taken from Ross (1953) with permission from the Company of Biologists.

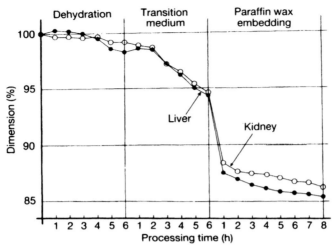

Figure 4.19:   Morphological changes of tissues during processing. A graph showing the linear shrinkage of tissue at each stage after fixation for dense, cellular tissues. Kidney and liver are given as examples; for explanation see text. Reproduced from Iwadare *et al.* (1984) with permission from the authors and the Royal Microscopical Society.

dration in alcohol (which as a fixative causes gross shrinkage) and takes place in particular at the beginning of immersion in the higher grades. The greatest amount of shrinkage (5–10%) is due to infiltration with hot paraffin wax, and takes place, similarly, at the beginning of immersion in wax. The effect of the transition media, in this case xylene or chloroform, is reported as 2–5%.

The effect of the transition medium on tissue morphometry is important, and is independent of the original fixative used to treat the tissue. Xylene is routinely used for cheapness, but causes the greatest shrinkage. Benzene shrinks less, and is quickly eliminated during embedding, but is highly carcinogenic. Dioxan shrinks to the same extent as xylene, and chloroform is intermediate. For research studies, or delicate tissues such as embryos, toluene or an essential oil (e.g. cedar-wood oil) should be used.

Similar results have also been published by Boonstra *et al.* (1983), who investigated cervical tissue. They looked in addition at the effect of fixation, concluding that 8% formalin fixation caused about 3% shrinkage, and that dehydration, clearing and embedding caused 12–15% shrinkage of the cervical tissue. Stowell (1941) came to similar conclusions, and also investigated the effect of different embedding procedures. Shrinkage can be reduced by embedding in nitrocellulose, and is less if the nitrocellulose is cold. Paraffin wax shrinks appreciably, by about 15% in volume, when it cools and exerts a compression effect on the tissue. Another particularly thorough study was carried out by Brain (1966). He measured and published silhouettes of mouse head profiles. Ethyl alcohol is a good dehydrant, better than other alcohols or acetone, but shows a large variation (7–16%) between dehydration and infiltration with wax. Methyl salicylate and methyl benzoate were better clearing agents (11–14% overall shrinkage) than xylene, chloroform or essential oils (29–34%).

The changes occuring in liver during processing into GMA resin have been reported by Handstede and Gerrits (1983). They found that 2–3 μm sections shrank during dehydration following fixation, and that this was greatest (9%) in 96% ethanol. Although there is no need to use a transition medium, the use of methyl benzoate does allow more reliable and reproducible sections to be cut from the block, and it can serve as a storage medium. The amount of shrinkage due to the use of methyl benzoate was 2%. During infiltration, unlike MMA, there is 2–5% swelling followed by 1–2% shrinkage of both MMA and GMA during polymerization. There is an enormous expansion of sections when they are stretched and dried, from 10–12% at 60°C to 13–15% at 20°C. The degree of stretching can be reduced by increasing the proportion of plasticizer in the resin mixture. Non-recoverable compression was about 0.5–1.0%; overall, therefore, plastic sections will suffer expansion of about 6% after drying onto the slide.

4.11 Sectioning difficulties

Tissues that are hard or friable or contain much blood and yolk, may disintegrate on cutting and floating out. Sections curl as they are cut, and are then flattened on water, but the flattening does not involve the same type of plastic flow, and transverse fractures can often be seen in friable material. They may be preserved either by using adhesive tape to capture each section, or by painting 0.5% celloidin in absolute alcohol, ether or acetone on the face of the block before each section is cut. The sections can be floated out in the normal way with the celloidin face up on a slightly hotter water-bath, and may present fewer folds if floated on 80% alcohol. If the tissue is very tough and hard, it may be difficult to cut, and the time in alcohol and clearing agents should be reduced to a minimum.

Friable tissues may benefit from not over-chilling and cutting with an increased rake angle. Connective tissue, particularly if inadequately processed, may absorb water, or else spring unduly as it is cut, tearing and disrupting the wax matrix. The best sections will be the transparent ones that come off first. Subsequent sections that have white areas should be discarded, since these are air spaces formed from the cracking of the tissue. Hard sections can be cut with a reduced rake angle, soaked with Mollifex for 30 min or one of the media listed below. Despite the use of cold block with Ralph knives, thin sections of skin can be difficult to cut. Nanchahal and Watts (1984) used a cryostat to cut 1 μm sections at −15°C, and cooled the wax gradually to this temperature to avoid cracking.

4.11.1 Softening fluids

Paraffin sections are usually softened with ice in freezer trays, such as are found in a domestic refrigerator. Where the specimens have just been blocked out, the ice serves to harden the paraffin prior to cutting.

Baker's fluid
This solution is especially good for those tissues which are either brittle and/or include friable tissue, such as blood clots.

60% ethyl alcohol	90 ml
Glycerol	10 ml

Where this mixture does not produce the necessary softening of very hard tissues, try Lendrum's fluid.

Lendrum's fluid

Glycerol	90 ml
Aniline	10 ml

Two or three days soaking with the block face down in a thin layer of fluid (a Petri dish is suitable) will allow most tissues to be cut to the extent that the fluid has penetrated. The mixture may discolour the wax, but this is not detrimental.

Foster and Gifford's fluid
This method is given for refractory plant material containing cellulose and lignin. Where the material is very hard to cut, use the protocol with a greater proportion of lactic acid.

Distilled water	36 ml
95% ethyl alcohol	54 ml
Lactic acid	10 ml
Distilled water	32 ml
95% ethyl alcohol	48 ml
Lactic acid	20 ml

Other workers recommend using 10% ammonium hydroxide, in a fume hood, for up to 30 min.

4.11.2 Static

Static occurs during sectioning as a result of friction, particularly in hot dry atmospheric conditions. The charged sections are often badly compressed and difficult to handle since they adhere to the microtome and handling instruments. Many technicians breathe, or 'huff', on the section as it comes off the knife to reduce curling and the effect of static. Other common measures to reduce static are to section in a room of low ambient temperature and of high humidity (place a bowl of boiling water next to the microtome), and to cool both block and knife. Grounding the microtome alone is not always effective, since the technician also acquires a static charge, which causes problems whilst handling the sections. Some authors advise cutting barefoot whilst touching a plate linked both to the microtome and earthed to ground! It is also possible to buy commercial antistatic guns that can be mounted in close proximity to the microtome, or within the chamber of the cryostat, to eliminate static.

4.11.3 Summary

The quality of the final section is influenced by:

(i)   The fixation and processing of the tissues.
(ii)   The type and hardness of the wax.
(iii) The quality, sharpness and the set of the knive.
(iv)   The speed of cutting.
(v)   The temperature of the block, environment and humidity.

The rake angle should be as large as possible, while the clearance angle should be as small as possible without fouling the block. The bevel and cutting angles and facet width should also be as small as possible to reduce section compression, without excessively increasing the radius of curvature of the knife, or amplitude of edge deflection. A cool knife, preferably etched, with a well-sharpened blade free from scratches and nicks is essential. Fault-diagnosis tables (*Tables 4.3* and *4.4*) are provided below to help solve problems with microtomy and cryotomy.

4.12 Vibratomes (tissue choppers)

Some histochemical techniques are carried out on fresh or fixed tissue which has not been frozen. Such tissue is usually embedded in agar or gelatin and cut under fluid (water or 0.1 M phosphate buffer pH 7.4, with or without saline). However, firm fibrous animal and botanical tissues may be cut without embedding—the fresh tissue being stuck directly onto the block. The thickness of sections cut with the vibratome, or tissue chopper, ranges from 20–200 μm, and it produces better thick sections of fixed material than the base-sledge microtome. There are several different types of tissue chopper manufactured: the H-1250 MicroCut (*Figure 4.20*), the Sorvall TC-2 Tissue Sectioner, the Jung VT 1000 and the Oxford Vibratome. These machines employ a continuously lubricated vibrating razor or custom-made disposable blade. The sections are manipulated with a curved seeker and brush, and transferred to fixative or holding buffer prior to staining. The blade vibrates in the horizontal plane, and advances over the tissue mounted on a stub which is held in a fixed chuck. Both the amplitude of vibration and the speed of advance can be altered, and the cutting action is in the form of a sine wave, which is lightly imprinted upon the surface of the gelatin block.

Table 4.3: Sectioning fault diagnosis

Fault	Cause	Remedy
Ribbon and consecutive sections are curved	Leading/trailing edges of block are not parallel	Trim parallel with sharp scalpel, and align block parallel with knife edge
	Knife blunt in one area	Sharpen knife or use new area of edge
	Surplus wax at one side	Trim away extra wax: care thick section
		Block not even temperature throughout
Alternate thick/thin sections (usually with compresssion of thin)	Wax soft. Knife/block loose	Cool block or re-embed tissue
	Insufficient clearance angle. Tilt too great	Tighten and adjust knife and/or block
	Faulty microtome	Check microtome for wear; apply oil
Parallel thick/thin zones (chattering)	Knife/block loose	Tighten adjustments, check for wear
	Knife tilt angle too steep	Reduce tilt angle
	Tissue/wax too hard (? a metallic note heard)	Use heavy knife, reduce slant
	Calcified areas	Use softening fluid. Decalcify tissue
Scores or splits in sections perpendicular to the knife edge	Nick in knife edge	Re-sharpen
	Hard particles in tissue	Decalcify, remove/dissect or use new tissue
	Hard particles in wax	Re-embed in fresh filtered wax
Sections won't ribbon	Wax too hard. Debris on knife edge	Breathe on block. Put soft wax on leading edge of block or re-embed
		Clean accretion off knife with xylene
	Tilt too steep/shallow	Adjust tilt angle of knife
	Cutting rate too slow	Increase rate and/or warm up room
Sections are attached to block on return	Insufficient clearance angle	Increase clearance angle
	Debris on knife/block edge	Clean debris/trim block, as above
	Static	Increase humidity, use burner to ionize air. Earth microtome; use static gun
Areas of tissue in block not present in sections	Incomplete processing and impregnation of tissue	Re-embed in last wax, or reprocess
	Tissue detaching from chuck	Re-attach with hot spatula to chuck

Table 4.3: *continued*

Fault	Cause	Remedy
Compression of sections	Blunt knife	Re-sharpen
	Knife bevel too great	Re-sharpen secondary facets or re-grind
	Wax too soft	Cool block or re-embed
	Cutting speed too fast	Reduce, especially for soft tissues
Sections expand and disintegrate on water of floatation bath	Poor impregnation of tissue	Re-impregnate in last wax under vacuum
	Water too hot	Cool water bath
Sections roll on knife	Knife blunt	Re-sharpen
	Tilt angle too great	Reduce knife tilt
	Insufficient rake angle	Re-grind shallower bevel angle
	Thickness set too large for (hard) wax in use	Reduce thickness, cool block; breathe on sections. Re-embed in softer wax
Sections crumble	Inter-medium (clearing agent) or alcohol not completely removed	Return to absolute alcohol, as for dehydrated tissues and re-process
	Wax too soft	Cool and/or re-embed in harder wax
	Knife is blunt	Re-sharpen knife
Resistance to knife is felt when block at lower limit of travel (rotary/rocker)	Insufficient clearance angle	Increase
Sections unevenly thick (metallic ring on cutting)	Tilt angle too great; a second section cut with feed disengaged, the block having expanded to original size	Reduce tilt
Sections have small irremovable wrinkles (present especially brain or lymph node)	Cutting is too fast/forceful	Cut with a slower and smoother stroke
Sections bulge in middle	Wax cool in centre, warm on outside. Central part of knife sharp. Hard wax/tissue in soft embedment	Let block temperature equilibrate after cooling
		Move knife
		Re-embed
	Residual clearing agent	
Object breaks away from wax; shattered by knife	Poor impregnation	Re-embed
	Tissue too hard	Soak to soften, embed in harder wax, double-embed or embed in resin
	Wrongly processed	Re-process, avoid xylene with muscle

Table 4.4:   Cryotomy fault diagnosis

Fault	Cause	Remedy
Poor morphology throughout tissue	Inadequate dissection Delay before dissection	Do not stretch, bend or chop, but slice tissue to cut. Freeze immediately, or perfuse fix with sucrose infusion
Holes in tissue	Large ice crystal formation or thawing/refreezing in cryostat	Rapidly freeze, use isopentane cooled by nitrogen. Use heat sink in body of cryostat chamber
'Fuzzy' morphology	Excess pressure on slide when picking up the section	Use less pressure
'Smeared' morphology	Lateral movement on pick-up	Lower slide without movement
Sections do not adhere to slide	Slides too cold or uncoated with adhesive	Warm slide locally with finger, or coat with adhesive
Sections scramble or blow away from knife edge when sectioning	Static electricity build-up	Earth posterior face of anti-roll plate Wipe plate with cold acetone Metal-coat anti-roll plate
Sections are scored perpendicular to knife edge	Dull knife edge	Sharpen. Should get 20–30 blocks of soft tissue per new edge, before knife needs replacing/resharpening
	Dirty leading edge of anti-roll plate	Clean edge of anti-roll plate
Tissue cracks as it is frozen	Tissue too thick Freezing too abrupt	Use smaller pieces Pre-cool chuck
Tissue breaks loose	Tissue too cold Trimming advance too great Freezing too prolonged Insufficient embedding	Trim < 10 mm. Let tissue and block holder warm up. Remount cold mass of block on fresh media without quenching Freeze to chuck within holder
Insufficient knife clearance angle	Dirt on chuck or embedment	Clean and pare away excess embedment Re-set clearance angle
Knife fails to cut	Mechanical fault	If no advance check feed advance limit or impedance from frost

Table 4.4: *continued*

Fault	Cause	Remedy
Tissue advances, but is not cut		Rewind. Check tissue is firm on block Tighten all adjustments. Check anti-roll plate is not protruding to foul tissue Examine tissue for high fat content Check no debris on front/back of knife
Sections roll up	Sections are too thick (opaque) Anti-roll plate fault	Cut thinner sections Check anti-roll plate not too far back Check tape on edges of anti-roll plate Reduce the angle of the anti-roll plate to the knife
Sections do not flatten	Anti-roll plate worn, dirty or not in the correct position above the knife	Clean and adjust anti-roll plate
Sections thaw onto knife		Cool knife and anti-roll plate, check alcohol for cleaning is not left on knife or plate
Sections stick to plate		Check and clean dirt, fat or previous section from the anti-roll plate
Sections skew to one side or are caught and puckered	Sections catching on debris, knife or anti-roll plate	Clean all items Re-trim mesa, so adequate support is given throughout cutting stroke
Sections score or split vertically		Clean knife of debris front or back Persistence—knife blunt or knicked Clean anti-roll plate
Sections incomplete in width	Anti-roll plate not parallel with knife over section range	Realign anti-roll plate
Sections incomplete in height	Compression	Clean and re-set anti-roll plate. Check for static. Try cutting thinner sections or at a cooler ambient temperature
Sections fissured parallel to knife edge	Fixed tissue prone Unfixed tissue too cold to cut	Soak fixed tissue in gum sucrose Allow tissue to 'warm up' in cabinet

Table 4.4: *continued*

Fault	Cause	Remedy
Knife squeaks	Obstruction	Knife too cold < −40 °C and/or blunt
Variable section thickness	Irregular advance due to ice on feed screw or ratchet	Defrost and clean Repair worn mechanical items
	Knife/block/tissue loose	Tighten adjustments and/or remount tissue
	Insufficient clearance	Check clearance angle
	Tissue expansion	Check cabinet temperature, don't wait too long between taking sections
Sections compress	Too much static	See above
	Debris/moisture/ice on knife or anti-roll plate	Clean
	Tilt too great or knife blunt	Adjust
	Angle of anti-roll plate to knife too much or insufficient	Adjust
Tissue shatters	Tissue too cold or dehydrated	
Sections crumble or do not form	Blunt knife, insufficient clearance angle. Knife tilt too great. Knife and anti-roll plate worn	Remedy as above
	Tissue dehydrated/dried out	Re-embed
Tissues shatter	Tissue too cold, cut too thickly or dried out	'Warm' tissue, cut thinner sections or re-embed

Trim the block to size and stick onto the stub with cyanoacrylate glue, using a cocktail stick. The height of the block should not exceed the base dimensions so that the block is prevented from 'wobbling' as it is cut. Conversely, if the tissue is only just above the junction of the block and stub, the glue can interfere with the cutting and prevent good sections from being obtained. The stub is locked into the jaws of the vice chuck with an Allen key. It is important to ensure that the stub is not placed too low in the chuck so that there is insufficient travel of the micrometer screw at the front of the machine. A double-edged razor blade is broken in half and inserted into the holder by pulling down the bar clip. It is important to chose a good quality blade, and to ensure that it is held firmly in the holder. The machine is operated by a toggle switch at the front: flick the switch forward to advance the blade, and backwards to reverse it once a section has been cut. Take care that the reverse is not operated too late, or the section just cut will be pushed off the stage holding the chuck, and be lost into the reservoir of lubricating fluid.

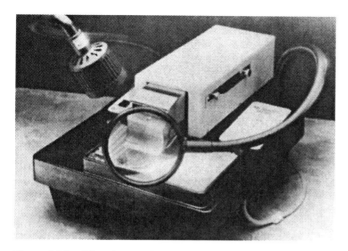

Figure 4.20: The tissue chopper. The H-1250 Micro-Cut, as an example, showing a disposable blade in position over a specimen on the circular stage. The blade may be advanced or retracted with the controls on the right; the stage is raised and lowered using the handwheel and micrometer feed screw on the right of the instrument. The frequency of the blade is operated using the controls on the left. The illuminated magnifying arm can be swung in or out as required (photograph courtesy of Energy Beam Sciences).

Once the blade has retracted over the block, move forward the microtome feed screw manually (calibrated in 1 µm steps) to the thickness of the next section, and advance the blade. The speed of advance and amplitude of vibration to suit the tissue being cut should be determined by trial and error. The speed of advance is usually more critical to producing good sections than amplitude, and must be precisely determined. As a general rule, the harder the tissue, the greater the speed and amplitude of vibration that is required to cut good sections, although if the amplitude is too great, the tissue sections are liable to fragment. Immersion in 2% bovine serum albumin between fixation and/or the addition of 0.3% borax to the embedding media may give a tougher block and obviate fragmentation. Further details of these procedures are given in Furness *et al.* (1977), Zelander and Kirkeby (1978) and Sallee and Russell (1993).

4.12.1 Macrotomes

Commercial food slicers have been used for sectioning soft organs with a large surface area (e.g. brains). Details of how to adapt a food slicer to section tough plant tissues has been reported by Lucansky (1976). The use of a macrovibratome for cutting thick (2 mm) sections of whole organs embedded in agar for further microscopic study has been reported by McLean and Prothero (1987).

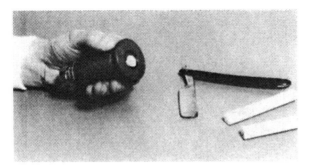

Figure 4.21:   The hand microtome. The pith sticks and traditional razor are to the right of the picture. Single-edged razor blades can also be used. A piece of pith is shown inserted in the microtome, although the well of this model will accept a larger diameter support. The knurled micrometer advance screw can be seen at the bottom of the instrument (the Mikrops manufactured by Flatters & Garnett).

4.13 Freehand sectioning

This method is simple, cheap, quick and easy but the results are not as good as the more sophisticated methods requiring expensive equipment. It is used primarily for botanical specimens where the tissue is refractory, and does not usually have to be hardened by prior fixation. Where tissues do have to be hardened, it is usually sufficient to store them for a day or two in 90% alcohol before cutting. The tissue is usually held either in elder pith (the European variety, *Sambucus nigra*, is better than the American species) or turgid *very fresh* carrot tissue. Elder pith can be stored in 70% alcohol, and cuts crisply, but expanded polystyrene has largely replaced the use of elder pith because it will not decay in storage and provides a firmer support than vegetable tissue matrices.

A hand microtome is shown in *Figure 4.21*. The pith must be cut, or carrot cylinders punched out, and trimmed to fit the microtome. The support cylinder is then slit longitudinally and the specimen wedged into it. The cylinder can then be bound up with thread or tape if needed, and the whole inserted into the microtome. It may pay to lubricate the inside of the microtome well, but *thinly*, with grease or low-melting point wax prior to inserting the specimen and block. Stems must be held in a tube of pith, carrot, polystyrene or wax. The well opens onto a platform of polished plate glass or metal, and a micrometer screw at the base advances the specimen and support block by 1–50 µm. It is possible to get sections as thin as 8 µm; the aim should be to cut routine sections at less than 12 µm.

Supporting tissues with pith or cork whilst using a sledge microtome has been advocated by Catling (1968) for sectioning partially dried, brittle, thin-walled aquatic plants. Thick (20–25 µm) sections were cut with a *very* sharp knife, which was flooded with 50% ethanol. The sections were then rapidly transferred to water to prevent collapse of the structure. Following bleaching, staining and partial dehydration, Catling recommends mounting in Euparal.

Tissues can also be supported embedded in wax or celloidin. The latter material is suitable, as sections must be at least 20 µm thick to cut properly. The material to be sectioned should be hardened by soaking in either 90% ethanol or fixative. Where a non-alcoholic fixative has been used the material should be transferred to 70% alcohol after fixation and any necessary washing. The sections are then embedded in celloidin to harden them, or are embedded in wax alone. Trim the material so that the transverse face is at right angles to the long axis, which should be about 1 cm long. Stand the block in the well of the microtome, and turn the advance screw so that the tissue lies below the cutting platform. Pour molten wax into the well (which now serves as a mould) and put it in the refrigerator to cool.

Advance the microtome screw so that the block can be trimmed and the tissue exposed for cutting. Trim the block so that the minimum amount of wax supports the tissue. Flood the blade with 70% alcohol or the appropriate storage fluid, and proceed to cut. The cutting stroke is best made with a large wedge profile razor that will sit flush on the platform, although a hollow ground instrument can be used. The razor blade should have an adequate handle, and be of shaving quality. Single-edged razor blades do not work satisfactorily with the hand microtome. The blade should be lubricated with storage fixative or 70% alcohol whilst cutting. Draw the blade across the tissue with a gentle yet firm oblique slicing stroke. Do not allow the resistance of the tissue to halt the cutting action of the blade. The sections should be lifted with a moist paint brush into fixative or 70% alcohol and stained by free-floating, or after mounting onto adhesive-coated slides.

References

Allison RT. (1978) The crystalline nature of histology waxes: a preliminary communication. *Med. Lab. Sci.* **35**, 355–363.

Allison R T. (1979) The crystalline nature of histology waxes: the effects of microtomy on the micro-structure of paraffin wax sections. *Med. Lab. Sci.* **36**, 359–372.

Anken RH, Kappel T. (1993) Orientation of small specimens for cryosectioning. *Biotechnic Histochem.* **68**, 305–307.

Anthony A, Colurso GJ, Bocan TMA, Doebler JA. (1984) Interferometric analysis of intrasection and intersection thickness variability associated with cryostat microtomy. *Histochem. J.* **16**, 61–70.

Bancroft JD. (1967) *An Introduction to Histochemical Technique.* Butterworths, London.

Bancroft JD. (1990) Frozen and related sections. In *Theory and Practice of Histological Techniques*, 3rd edn (eds JD Bancroft and A Stevens). Churchill Livingstone, Edinburgh, pp. 81–92.

Banthorpe MJ, Court RA. (1970) A substitute for the Shandon-Elliot lapping bar. *J. Med. Lab. Technol.* **27**, 446.

Barthel LK, Raymond PA. (1990) Improved method for obtaining 3 μm cryosections for immunocytochemistry. *J. Histochem. Cytochem.* **38**, 1383–1388.

Bennett HS, Wyrick AD, Lee SW, McNeil Jr JH. (1976) Science and art in preparing tissues embedded in plastic for light microscopy with special reference to glycol methacrylate, glass knives and simple stains. *Stain Technol.* **51**, 71–97.

Boonstra H, Oosterhuis JW, Fleuren GJ. (1983) Cervical tissue shrinkage by formaldehyde fixation, paraffin wax embedding, section cutting and mounting. *Virchows Arch. [Pathol. Anat.]* **402**, 195–201.

Brain EB. (1966) *The Preparation of Decalcified Sections.* Thomas, Springfield.

Butcher RG. (1971) The chemical determination of section thickness. *Histochemie* **28**, 131–136.

Butler JK. (1979) Methods for improved light microscope microtomy. *Stain Technol.* **54**, 53–69.

Catling DM. (1968) Preparing microtome sections of aquatic plants without embedding. *Proc. R. Microscop. Soc.* **3**, 126–128.

Clayden EC. (1971) *Practical Section Cutting and Staining*, 5th edn. Churchill Livingstone, Edinburgh.

Collins EM. (1969) Improved paraffin sectioning with etched microtome knife edges. *Stain Technol.* **44**, 33–37.

Culling CFA, Allison RT, Barr WT. (1985) *Cellular Pathology Technique*, 4th edn. Butterworths, London.

Dempster WT. (1942a) The mechanics of paraffin sectioning by the microtome. *Anatom. Record* **84**, 241–267.

Dempster WT. (1942b) Distortions due to the sliding microtome. *Anatom. Record* **84**, 269–274.

Feeney JF. (1944) The rapid preparation of celloidin serial sections following India ink injections. *Stain Technol.* **19**, 137–140.

Fink S. (1992) A solvent-free coating-procedure for the improved preparation of cryostat sections in light microscope histochemistry. *Histochemistry* **97**, 243–246.

Furness JB, Costa M, Blessing WW. (1977) Simultaneous fixation and production of catecholamine fluorescence in central nervous tissue by perfusion with aldehydes. *Histochem. J.* **9**, 745–750.

Godkin SE, Knight GE. (1975) A supplementary sliding microtome vise for small sections. *Stain Technol.* **50**, 62.

Gray SJ. (1972) *Essentials of microtomy.* Butterworths, London.

Handstede JG, Gerrits PO. (1983) The effects of embedding in water-soluble plastics on the final dimensions of liver sections. *J. Microsc.* **131**, 79–86.

Helander KG. (1983) Thickness variations within individual paraffin and glycol methacrylate sections. *J. Microsc.* **132**, 223–227.

Helander KG. (1984) The Ralph knife in practice. *J. Microsc.* **135**, 139–146.

Iwadare T, Mori H, Ishiguro K, Takeishi M. (1984) Dimensional changes of tissues in the course of processing. *J. Microsc.* **136**, 323–327.

Ishii T, Kasama K, Kondo M. (1990) Improvement of the quality of frozen sections from formalin fixed tissue. *Stain Technol.* **65**, 43–44.

Johansson O. (1983) The vibratome–Ralph knife combination: a useful tool for immunhistochemistry. *Histochem. J.* **15**, 265–273.

Lamb RA. (1973) Waxes for Histology. In *Histopathology: Selected Topics* (ed. HC Cook). Bailliere-Tindall, London, pp. 123–146.

Lange PW, Engström A. (1954) Determination of thickness of microscopic objects. *Lab. Invest.* **3**, 116–131.

Lucansky TW. (1976) The macrotome: a new approach to sectioning large plant specimens. *Stain Technol.* **51**, 199–201.

McLean M, Prothero J. (1987) Coordinated three-dimensional reconstruction from serial sections at macroscopic and microscopic levels of resolution: the human heart. *Anatom. Record* **219**, 434–439.

Merriam RW. (1957) Determination of section thickness in quantitative microspectrophotometry. *Lab. Invest.* **6**, 28–43.

Nanchahal J, Watts RH. (1984) A procedure for cutting one micrometer sections of wax embedded skin. *Stain Technol.* **59**, 53–55.

Pearse AD. (1973) The sharpening of Jung K microtome knives with particular reference to cryostat sectioning. *Med. Lab. Technol.* **30**, 117–122.

Pearse AD, Marks R. (1974) Measurement of section thickness in quantitative microscopy with special reference to enzyme histochemistry. *J. Clin. Pathol.* **27**, 615–618.

Pearse AGE. (1980) *Histochemistry: Theoretical and Applied*, Vol I, 4th edn. Churchill Livingstone, Edinburgh.

Powell, A Murgatroyd LB. (1970) A new technique for sharpening microtome knives. *J. Med. Lab. Technol.* **27**, 79–82.

Reid N, Beesley JE. (1991) *Sectioning and Cryosectioning for Electron Microscopy*, Practical Methods in Electron Microscopy, Vol. 13 (ed. AM Glauert), Elsevier, Amsterdam.

Richards PR. (1984) An anti-roll plate system for Ralph knives. *J. Microsc.* **133**, 185–190.

Ross KFA. (1953) Cell shrinkage caused by fixatives and paraffin wax embedding in ordinary cytological preparations. *Q. J. Microscop. Sci.* **94**, 125–139.

Sallee CJ, Russell DF. (1993) Embedding of neural tissue in agarose or glyoxyl agarose for vibratome sectioning. *Biotechnic Histochem.* **68**, 360–368.

Schrader RM, Zeman FJ. (1971) Cryostat sectioning: modification of the antiroll plate. *Stain Technol.* **46**, 275–278.

Semba R. (1979) Contributions to semithin sectioning on a conventional rotary microtome. *Stain Technol.* **54**, 251–255.

Smith A. (1962) Tissue shrinkage caused by attachment of paraffin sections to slides: its effects on staining. *Stain Technol.* **37**, 339–345.

Stowell RE. (1941) Effect on tissue volume of various methods of fixation, dehydration and embedding. *Stain Technol.* **16**, 67–83.

Szczesny TM. (1978) Holder assembly for 'Ralph' type glass knives. *Stain Technol.* **53**, 50–51.

Turner G, Novacky A. (1973) Mounting and quenching thin leaves for cryostat sectioning. *Stain Technol.* **48**, 263–265.

Viebahn C, Lüttenberg H-P. (1989) A modified anti-roll plate as a remedy for the ill-effects of electrical charge during sectioning. *J. Histochem. Cytochem.* **37**, 1157–1160.

Vincent JFV. (1991) Automating the microtome. *Microsc. Anal.* **23**, 19–21.

Watkins S. (1991) Insight into hybridization and immunohistochemistry. In *Current Protocols in Molecular Biology*, Vol. 2 (eds FM Ausubel, R Brent, RE Kingston *et al.*), pp. 14. 01–14. 613. Greene Publishing Associates, Inc. and John Wiley & Sons, Inc., New York.

Zelander T, Kirkeby S. (1978) Vibratome sections of difficult tissues. *Stain Technol.* **53**, 251–255.

Zheng-Yi W. (1993) A new antiroll device for cryostat wax sectioning. *Biotechnic Histochem.* **68**, 38–41.

5 Other Preparative Methods

This chapter gives a further selection of methods, as alternatives to the thin sectioning described in the previous chapter. Specimens other than sliced tissue are found as free cells or disaggregated tissue, or else as entire organisms which may be mounted in dry or fluid form. The various ways by which each of these different types of material may be made into suitable preparations are dealt with in turn. This handbook does not give protocols for preserving and preparing every specimen for microscopical examination, but deals with the principles of microtechnique. For specific protocols and methods suited to different taxonomic groups of organisms, the reader is referred to Guyer (1953), Gray, P. (1964), Bradbury (1973), Wagstaffe and Fidler (1955, 1968) and Marson (1983). An excellent text for microbiology, which has stood the test of time, is Collins *et al.* (1989).

5.1 Cytological methods

Thin sectioning allows the investigator to study the relationship of cell shape and inter-related position, which is often crucial for diagnosis or research, but this method requires drastic biopsy techniques (often under anaesthaesia) or killing of the experimental animal involved. For large subjects, in particular humans, it is often preferential to collect samples of cells either by fine needle aspiration biopsy (FNAB) or in secretions. Alternatively, cytological examination can be made of cells exfoliated into body fluids.

FNABs are taken using an 18–23 gauge needle (0.6–1.2 mm diameter) and a 3, 5 or 10 ml syringe, as suited to the size of the lesion. Where the sample is diluted by blood, it should be concentrated according to the method of Abele *et al.* (1985) or fixed in a lysing fixative. Erythrocytes can be lysed with 3% acetic acid added to the 95% ethanol, with Carnoy's or Clarke's fixative or by brief immersion for 1 min in 2 M urea after fixation in 95% ethanol. The reader is referred to Boon and Drijver (1986), Coleman and Chapman (1989) and Orell *et al.* (1992), for detailed assessments of the techniques involved in the collection of clinical specimens by scraping, aspiration or exfoliation.

Cytological specimens are collected unfixed, and therefore must be treated as potentially infectious. Unless the specimens are so small that they dry immediately or are otherwise intended to be dry-fixed for Romanowsky-Giemsa (R-G) staining, they must be wet-fixed as soon as possible after collection. Where cells are dry-fixed, this must be rapid, otherwise impaired staining and morphology will result. Air-dried samples must be fixed in 100% methanol for at least 5 min, after which they can be stained or stored. Where it is possible to transport slides in secure containers, use 95% ethyl alcohol as a transport medium; most cells adhere well to the slide because of their mucoprotein content. For cells less likely to adhere (e.g. watery samples), use an aerosol spray or apply the fixative at a lower concentration using a dropper bottle. It is not a good idea to re-use fixative solutions, as they may contain floating cells which can cross-transfer between specimens.

As pointed out in Chapter 1, the constitution of the sample and structure of cells differs between cytology and histology (see *Figure 1.3*). Fatty and immature cells are likely to lose their cytoplasm, and squamous cells, which may appear columnar in thin section, lie on their large side to appear flat in a cytological preparation. Staining will tend to be more uneven in cytological preparations, since whole cells and clumps, rather than a thin plane of tissue, are present in the sample.

5.2 Cytological fixatives

The most usual fixatives are the alcohols ethanol and methanol. Formaldehyde is not used so widely in cytology as in histology. The strength of the initial fixative is often quite low, to allow cell adherence to the slide. The most common fixative is 95% ethanol; the addition of 3% acetic acid will improve the fixation of nucleoprotein and promote lysis of erythrocytes. Where the percentage strength is less than 70%, post-fixation is recommended, and is necessary for air-dried material. Other fixatives that may be used in place of 95% ethanol are 100% methanol (usually following fixation by air-drying) and 80% propan-2-ol. Methanol, when used prior to R-G staining, must be acetone and formalin free. The propan-2-ol is used at 80% strength because the neat alcohol causes more shrinkage than ethanol, and the water counteracts this effect. Since it is illegal in many countries to send fixing fluids via the post, spray fixative mixtures of ethanol and PEG (Carbowax) are used. The PEG provides a protective layer to prevent the sample drying out, and must be removed using two rinses of 95% ethanol (5–10 min each) before subsequent treatment.

Samples to be stained by Papanicolaou's stain must be wet-fixed for at least 20 min, and not air-dried. Fixation which has been hurried will result in blurred chromatin and pale, inadequate staining. Where wax from spray fixation is carried over into the staining solutions, nuclei appear foggy lacking detail, and cytoplasm stains pale blue. If there is a danger that smears will dry out before fixation (particularly where little mucus is present), the slide should be moistened or sprayed with fixative, and the spray or container should be made ready for immediate use after taking the preparation. Good spraying is a matter of practice to ensure that cells are impregnated, yet not saturated on the slide. The ideal distance is from 7.5–15 cm (3–6") for non-aerosols and 15–25 cm (6–10") for aerosol sprays; one should aim to spray an even layer of fixative in a single pass that leaves a very thin layer of wax on the slide. Because of the loss of floating cells, and the green background seen with wet-fixed Papanicolaou-stained smears on gelatinized slides, Kung *et al.* (1989) cytocentrifuge concentrated cell populations onto albumen slides and air-dry these. The air-dried slides are then rehydrated in 0.9% sodium chloride for 30 sec, fixed in 95% ethanol and stained with haematoxylin and eosin (H & E).

5.3 Cytocentrifuging and sedimentation

The Shandon Cytospin III is a specially designed instrument which spins a cell suspension onto a microscope slide clipped under a filter which removes the diluent. Up to 12 slides can be spun at one time, and the instrument contains a removable enclosed rotor which permits infectious material to be treated. *Figure 5.1* shows the Cytospin and sample chamber assembly which holds the slide and filter in the rotor. Trial and error will show the best cell concentration and speed to use; but a 100 μl aliquot of 10^6 cells ml^{-1} spun at 20 000 g for 5 min is a suitable starting point. Moistening the filter paper before centrifugation with saline, and limiting the diluent volume to 500 μl, will give optimum yields of cells.

Where there are very few cells in the sample, Duarte (1991) suggests preparing a pellet by centrifugation, embedding by freezing in Tissue-Tek or similar medium, and fixing the pellet. Following plastic embedding, the cell block will then yield many sections from an initially scanty sample. Duarte recommends an ultracentrifugation step of 30 000 g for 3 min, which should be used with caution, as many cell types will suffer morphological disruption at this centrifugal force. As a general rule, a maximum of 700 g for spinning cells in a watery diluent should be adhered to. Cells from paraffin-embedded tissues may be examined as monolayers. This procedure (van Driel-Kulker *et al.*, 1987) is useful where fresh material is difficult to obtain; and permits retrospective studies of selected material.

The cytocentrifuge is excellent for preparing very thin samples of cells, but the forces used can be sufficiently violent to cause damage and distortion, particularly to unfixed cells and those with delicate processes. An alternative method (Boon and Drijver, 1986) for preparing samples is

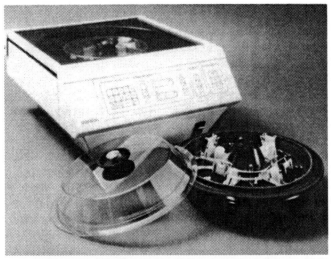

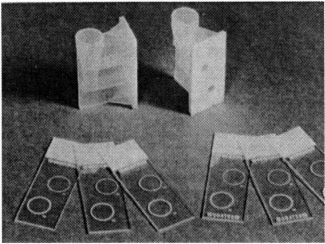

Figure 5.1: The cytocentrifuge. The Shandon Cytospin® 3 is shown (top) with the removable rotor and lid. The rotor contains four spring-clip assemblies which contain the filter papers and slides as one unit. The bottom picture shows the Cytofunnel disposable single-use units, suitable for infectious specimens. The custom-made slides which are also shown are not essential, but their white circles aid location of the specimen (photographs courtesy of Shandon, Life Sciences International).

shown in *Figure 5.2*. A cylindrical 300 g brass weight with a central bore holds a filter with a suitably sized hole over a microscope slide. The filter can be made from blotting paper with a cork borer or hole punch, or from a wire mesh (Cobb *et al.*, 1990). Support the apparatus on a stand (to prevent flooding the microscope slide) within a Petri dish. Pour the cell suspension into the central bore of the weight. Since fixed cells flatten and

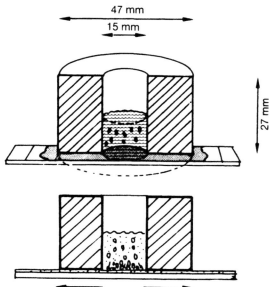

Figure 5.2: Cell sedimentation. Sedimentation using van der Griendt's method. The dimensions of the 300 g brass weight are given. Mucoid material should be strained through a tea-strainer into the centre of the weight. The residue can then be smeared by one of the methods outlined in *Figure 5.3*. Reproduced from Boon and Drijver (1985) with permission from Macmillan Press Ltd.

adhere less well to the slide than if unfixed or centrifuged, care should be taken during post-fixing and subsequent treatment against gross cell loss.

Filters can also be used to concentrate cells using a Büchner funnel and water vacuum pump. A polycarbonate filter with a pore size of 5 µm is suitable, and the cells should be post-fixed in 95% ethanol for 30–60 min. Do not use absolute ethanol or methanol, which will soften the membrane. After staining, take the filter briefly through isopropyl alcohol (propan-2-ol), then 95% ethanol, and mount in sufficient mountant to prevent air bubbles. Imprints can be made from filters onto adhesive-coated slides, or those cooled to –20°C.

5.3.1 Adherence and loss of cells

It is important to take acount of the factors which determine selective cell loss, particularly in the clinical diagnosis of suspected carcinomas. For example, during sedimentation, larger (malignant) cells overlie the smaller cells, and are more easily lost. This loss may be enhanced by the type of fixative used and the rate of fixation. Non-alcoholic fixatives (formol-saline) fix slowly, and therefore (unlike alcohols) mucoprotein is not coagulated fast into an adhesive mesh. The surface tension forces present when changing fluids may lift cells off a slide; use well-mixed fluids and graded alcohols to minimize this effect. The factors which influence

Table 5.1: Factors influencing the adherence of cells to slides

Promotion of adherence	Loss of adherence
Non-fixation (cells are softer)	Wet fixation
Fixation by air-drying	Premature washing (saline)
	Watery sample (e.g. urine)
Retention of mucus and protein	Non-alcoholic fixatives (formol-saline) fix slowly: mucoprotein not coagulated
Use of an adhesive (or etch with silane)	Use of smooth glass
	Increased viscosity of sample
Applying PEG as 'glue' (cells remain adherent after removal)	Surface tension currents of alcohol/water phases during dehydration
Use of frozen slides	
Centrifugation	Absorbtion by cytocentrifuge filter
Larger cells have greater surface area	Sedimentation: large cells overlie smaller ones, and are more easily lost

the adherence of cells to the slide are listed in *Table 5.1*. Carbowax (2%), bovine serum albumin or fetal calf serum can be added to the cell deposit to promote adhesion before smearing. Alternatively, the smear can be coated with LVN (Section 7.7.1) to prevent cell loss.

5.4 Smears

The simplest way to collect cells is by scraping or brushing them from the site of interest, and making a smear on a slide. Smears can also be made directly from aspirates, or first concentrated as a pellet or onto the slide.

The aim of smearing is to get a *very thin* preparation, which takes some practice. Semi-solid tissue can be smeared by rotating a small amount of material between two slides or the coverslip and slide. Alternatively, the material is pulled between two slides (*Figure 5.3*). Another way is to deposit a small suspension of material onto the slide, and brush it from the centre outwards down the slide in an elongated spiral using a spatula or swab.

5.5 Imprints and replicas

These methods lie between cytological and histological methods, since individual cells can be examined, yet their spatial relationship within the tissue is to some extent preserved. Fresh tissue can be trimmed flat on one face, and pressed onto a slide without any lateral movement. The process should be repeated on each slide, since the first imprint often contains excess fluid and blood. Fat should be trimmed to a minimum, or avoided,

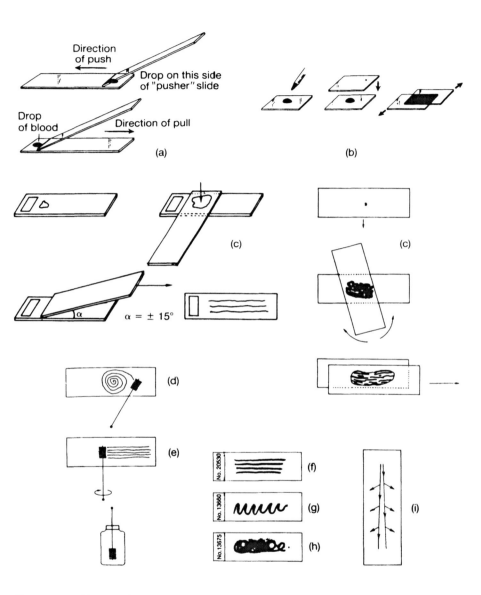

Figure 5.3: Methods for smearing cells. Nine methods of making smears. Pushing a drop of fluid (e.g. blood) between two slides (a) is the best-known technique. Samples prepared on a coverslip can be pulled from a drop (b). Aspirates containing thicker elements (e.g. sputum, mucus) may best be prepared using a combination of both these techniques (c). The material is first squashed then pulled into a smear using a second slide. Fluid material may also be smeared from brushes or swabs. For preparations to be wet-fixed (speed is essential to prevent drying!) use the circular method (d); those to be dry-fixed are best smeared by rolling the brush in a continuous line over the slide (e). Gynaecological specimens, or others taken with a spatula may be smeared horizontally (f), in a zig-zag (g), clockwise (h) or fish-tail (i). Adapted from Boon and Drijver (1985), and Davenport (1960) *Histological and Histochemical Technics*, with permission from Macmillan Press Ltd and Saunders College Publishing, respectively.

since it tends to smudge the final result. The amount of pressure will vary according to the type of tissue and its pathological state. Benign tissue requires much firmer pressure than malignant lesions. A comparison of the diagnostic value of the imprint technique compared with conventional histological methods has been reported by Tribe (1965) and Lee (1982). Although fat tends to give a poor quality result, blocks of fat can be imprinted onto a silanized slide and briefly washed to provide a fresh, easily prepared, positive control for fat staining techniques. This method obviates the need to cut and keep frozen sections for controls.

Replication can be used to examine the exposed surface of tough, herbaceous tissues without the need for sectioning (Balasubramanian, 1979). This is useful where maceration and sectioning of such tissues may preclude morphometric analysis. The surface to be replicated should be swabbed with 70% ethanol and blotted dry to remove as much surface moisture as possible. A solution of polystyrene (e.g. DPX thickened by partial evaporation of the xylene solvent) or clear nail varnish is painted onto the surface and allowed to dry. Once dry, the film can be incised and lifted free with a piece of transparent cellophane tape which is then inverted onto a slide. For precise work, where the microscope objective must be used with a coverslip of known thickness (Section 7.6), the tape (with the replica uppermost) is stuck to a coverslip which is then mounted in the usual way.

5.5.1 Cell blocks

The cell block also occupies an intermediate position between cytology and histology. It may be advantageous to concentrate cells, fix and entrap them in a 5% agar mesh for examination (e.g. for intra-cytoplasmic antigens or clinical diagnoses) by thin sectioning. Temporary cell blocks can be frozen by re-suspension of the deposit in a drop of embedding compound which is then snap-frozen in liquid nitrogen and sectioned in the normal way. This technique lends itself particularly well to coelemic and serous effusions (which clot) and mucoid tissue.

The mucus present (e.g. in sputum samples) should be liquefied before fixation by blending, ultrasonication or shaking with Tween 80 followed by centrifugation at $700\,g$ for 5 min. The pellet is fixed in 95% ethanol, 10% formol-saline or picro-alcohol fixative (13 g of picric acid in 70% ethanol) overnight. Alternatively, samples can be microwave-fixed (2–5 min in 10% formalin). The pellet is re-suspended in heated agar (melting point 98°C) cooled to 50°C, centrifuged at $700\,g$ for 3 min and processed, once set (below 40°C), as described in Chapter 3. Some workers (Kok *et al.*, 1986), prefer to fix, dehydrate and embed the samples for cell blocks using microwaves. This technique is not only rapid, but is safer and gives superior results. A study on the effectiveness of cell blocks, as opposed to smears, for clinical diagnosis has been published by Gray, B. (1964).

5.6 Squashes

Squashing is used for material that is just too hard for smearing, but cannot be sectioned without embedding. It is generally used for rapidly growing plant material such as root tips and anthers. Squashing differs from smearing in that tissue which requires squashing must usually be pretreated by maceration to remove the pectic middle lamella binding the cellulose walls of adjacent cells together.

The classic way to study chromosomes is to prepare a squash of a cell culture (Brocklehurst, 1993) arrested in metaphase by the mitotic inhibitor colchicine, and stain the chromosomes to show the distinctive shape and banding pattern by which they are karyotyped. There are different protocols according to the type of material used, but preparations are commonly made from peripheral blood leucocytes, insects and plant material, all of which are easily available. For further details concerning chromosome banding, the reader is referred to Sumner (1989).

5.6.1 Maceration

This technique is useful for dense or refractory materials which would otherwise obscure the protoplasm in the fresh state. Refer to Section 3.21 for the associated technique of selectively clearing plant tissue to enhance the structures of interest. Leaf tissue that is to be macerated should first be soaked in 95% ethanol to remove the chlorophyll. Shavings should be taken of harder material, to present a large surface area to the macerating fluid, and to allow the tissue to be teased out flat and subsequently mounted. Maceration is usually continued for 12–24 h, or until the edges of the tissue begin to fray visibly. The specimen should then be washed gently in running water for 2 h before staining and mounting. Maceration can be performed with enzymes on frozen sections, or using acids or alkalis. Humason (1972) recommends using one of the following.

2% aqueous chromic acid for 24 h or longer.
20% aqueous nitric acid for 24 h or longer.
Boric acid, saturated (6%) in sea water for marine forms with two drops of Lugol's iodine (1% iodine in 2% (aq) potassium iodide) per 25 ml, for 2–3 days.
33% aqueous potassium hydroxide for isolating smooth and striated muscle, for 1–2 h.

Herbaceous tissues, where the middle lamella is composed of pectin, can be macerated in 25% 2 M hydrochloric acid in 95% ethanol, while Schulze's fluid (0.5% potassium nitrate in concentrated nitric acid) is useful for woody specimens where the middle lamella is lignified and more resistant to maceration. These are not fixing solutions, so some form of fixation is usually required after maceration. Jeffrey's fluid (10% (aq) nitric acid and 10% (aq) chromic acid in equal parts) will fix in addition to macerating the tissue. Wash well before proceeding further.

5.7 Temporary mounts

Temporary mounts are useful for quick examination, for example to check a sample in the course of collection or permanent preparation. The simplest way to examine most material is merely to enclose a drop of fluid under a coverslip, which will be held in place by capillary attraction. Cells and fine particulate material can be suspended in water or physiological saline. Botanical tissues can be mounted for examination in 30% alcohol. Glycerol (30–50%) is useful in both cases where delicate objects may be damaged by manipulation, but the material should be washed in distilled water prior to making the preparation.

Small organisms can be enclosed (wet or dry) in a ring built up from layers of shellac or varnish. Larger objects can be placed in an aluminium cell cemented to a slide kept for temporary mounts. All that is required is for the top of the ring or cell to be moistened with water or glycerol and a coverslip lowered into place. With care, this method is also suitable for the examination of powders, pollen or Foraminifera. An alternative is to raise the coverslip clear of the object using Plasticine or small slips of thin card or plastic.

The traditional way in which temporary cell suspensions are examined is as a hanging drop. The inherent disadvantage of this method is that the suspended material quickly accumulates at the curved surface, which is not only difficult to focus on, but is particularly susceptible to vibration— an important point when examining specimens in the field. The lying drop obviates all these disadvantages, and also permits slides of machined aluminium or other non-breakable material to be used. If a metal slide with a central hole of suitable diameter is used, it is an easy matter to fix a coverslip to the slide with a smear of wax melted with a match or lighter. The sample can quickly be examined in the well so formed, which can be dismantled, cleaned and re-made in a few minutes.

5.7.1 Irrigation

Where it is helpful to study the effect of a changing environment on small organisms or living cells, the technique of irrigation should be considered. In its simplest form fluid is drawn under the coverslip from one side to another using blotting paper. If the stage is inclined, a glass slide with a strip 75 × 0.25 mm can be used to retain the fluid (*Figure 5.4*). Alternatively, the cells can be studied as a drop in a perfusion chamber (Dick, 1955) requiring at the minimum only a few millilitres of irrigation fluid.

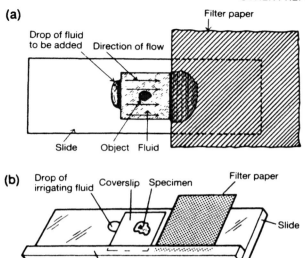

Figure 5.4: Irrigating preparations. Two methods of irrigating a preparation: (a) on a horizontal stage, (b) on an inclined stage. Reproduced from Bradbury (1973) with permission from Edward Arnold.

A more sophisticated design has been published by Pentz and Hörler (1992); this permits cell culture, and allows good resolution of fine detail, which is not always the case with tissue culture plastic (*Figure 5.5*). A further design of perfusion chamber, which permits temperature regulation of the cells or tissue, has been published by Sevcik *et al.* (1993).

5.8 Preparations of whole mounts in cells or 'boxes'

These types of preparation are used where the object does not need to be examined under high power. Small shells, Foraminifera, insect scales, mosses and dried plants (which are not subject to further decay) are examples of dry-mounted specimens; hydrated organisms and tissues (such as insects and nematode whole mounts) as well as aquatic organisms and cultures are usually preserved as fluid mounts. Partially stripped layers of intestines, block-stained to demonstrate the nervous sytem, may usefully be prepared as whole mounts (Costa *et al.*, 1980).

Where possible, the preparation should be mounted in a resin, which provides mechanical strength and stability against decomposition, and a higher refractive index for improved contrast and resolution. This is not

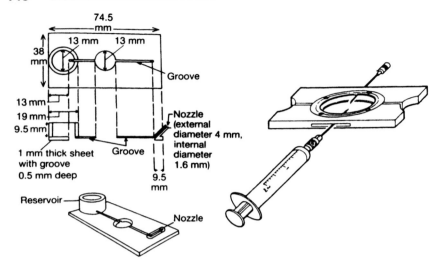

Figure 5.5: Tissue culture chambers. Left: simple design. Reproduced from Dick (1955) with permission from The Company of Biologists Ltd. Right: commercially available design. Reproduced from Pentz and Hörler (1992) with permission from the authors and The Royal Microscopical Society.

always possible, however, either because the tissue cannot withstand fixing and hardening, or because the dye stain is soluble in the dehydration or transition media. Glycerol is, therefore, an alternative choice, but cells containing this fluid are very difficult to seal; it should be avoided where aqueous gum media can be employed, or the preparation made with glycerin jelly. Like glycerol, glycerin jelly is of higher refractive index than purely aqueous mounts, and so displays greater contrast.

5.8.1 Dry mounts

The objects are contained within a cell composed of slide, coverglass and spacing ring, which is made up using a ringing table as described below and in Chapter 7. Aluminium or plastic rings are fixed onto the slide with gold-size, which is the best adhesive available for fine work, but is slow-drying. Modern glass adhesives can also be used and allowed to cure in the sun or under UV light, but these are thick, tricky to apply, and the ringing brush is difficult to clean.

Gold-size has the advantage that the glassware does not have to be chemically clean for good adhesion. It is usually sufficient to clean the slides with a good scouring powder, followed by a wash in water. Alternatively, a suitable adhesive is commercially available from Northern Biological Supplies (NBS).

Aluminium or plastic rings can be cut with a fine hacksaw from tubing in a mitre board (parting off in a lathe is better), and the excess swarf removed with emery paper. These rings—for constructing cells—can also be bought, either loose or fixed to slides, and are better than any rings made of bookbinder's millboard which can never be properly sealed and permit the growth of fungi and moulds.

The gold-size should be that sold for microscopical use made up in toluene. Gold-size sold for bookbinding and gilding is not suitable. To construct a cell, a suitable ring of gold-size should be turned onto the slide and allowed to dry. Apply a similar coat to the underside of the cell. Apply further coats to each surface and allow to dry for a few seconds until tacky. Press the cell onto the slide, and either clamp together with another slide held in place over the cell with a strong rubber band, or weight the cell down with a suitable weight. Leave the slide to dry for 3 days. At the end of this time inspect the seal for any air holes, which would later let in airborne microbes, and seal these if necessary. Do this by inspecting the undersurface of the cell and slide; where the glass specularly reflects the light, the seal is imperfect, and will have to be remade. The seal should be entirely matt in appearance. Scrape out the internal seepage of cement, but leave the outer seal. Do not use a solvent to wipe the inner seal, as for fluid mounts, as this may loosen the cell.

Black backgrounds can be provided for opaque specimens in one of two ways. A suitably sized piece of paper can be punched or cut out to fit the cell, and stuck into place with spray or fluid glue. Alternatively, NBS Matt Black Background, or a similar matt varnish (e.g. Humbrol® model enamel paint) can be used to paint the inside of the cell, but the 'rings' need practice to turn in a neat fashion. Several workers have used self-adhesive paper circles successfully. Ideally, the objects should be stuck on with a cement that has been incorporated into the matt black used to paint the cell.

Gum tragacanth can be bought from health shops as a powder or ready made up from NBS. The powder should be dissolved into twice its volume of 5% alcohol in distilled water to form a very thick jelly stock. This stock stores well; when required, mix a brushful into 1 ml water. The alcohol preservative leaves no residue, unlike phenol or thymol, but does require periodic replenishing. The glue is invisible in Canada balsam, and almost so in a dry mount. Gum tragacanth is only useful for sticking down very small objects, such as diatoms, small Foraminifera or insect scales. It does not have to be heated. Turn a *very* thin layer of gum tragacanth onto the bottom of the cell, and allow it to dry for a few minutes. Arrange the objects as required and breathe very carefully over the preparation. The warm moist air will cause the objects to stick firmly into the gum layer, with sufficient time to manoeuvre them before the gum tragacanth dries. Other cements may be found in Gray (1954).

Where Foraminifera are to be arranged on an opaque paper surface with gum tragacanth, they can be kept in place with a small amount of gum tragacanth applied with an eyelash probe. The specimen is manipulated using half a cocktail stick slit at the blunt end, with an eyelash inserted and held in place by glue or dental wax. It often helps to slice off the pointed tip of the eyelash with a scalpel so that a minute drop of adhesive can more easily be picked up and applied to the slide. Using a stereo or dissecting microscope, select a Foram and place it onto the drop of gum. If this drop is dry, do not moisten it, but place a futher drop of gum on top and place the object on that. Gum tragacanth will not adhere to a waxy or resinous surface, which may preclude some botanical specimens from this technique. For these use gold-size, but allow a few days to dry. Drops of gold-size or a modern contact adhesive can be used to stick large objects to the slide or paper circle insert.

Most biological samples contain water, and this must be removed before the dry mount is sealed. When making mounts of sand or insoluble particulate material, the samples can be washed and dehydrated simultaneously by rinsing in water followed by two washes in IMS or propan-2-ol. Botanical specimens should initially be dried between layers of blotting paper bound between stiff card to prevent shrivelling and curling. This initial drying should be fairly rapid, and no more than a few hours, to prevent discoloration of the sample, and is followed by a thorough drying in a dessicator, or warm, dust-free atmosphere. Silica gel is suitable for dessication (which can be enhanced under a light vacuum); this dessicant turns from bright blue to pink once it is exhausted, and can easily be re-charged by heating for a few minutes on high power in a microwave oven.

Once mounted, the preparations should be allowed to dry overnight in a dessicator, *dry* airing cupboard or similar warm environment. A thin ring of gold-size should be turned onto the top of the cell and a coverslip placed on top. It is a good idea to use a thick coverslip (No. 2 or 3) where objectives of low numerical aperture will be used, as this offers greater stability to the cell. The preparation should not be too warm when the coverslip is applied, or else air contraction will spoil the preparation as the gold-size is drawn in. Run around the top of the coverslip with a pair of blunt forceps to seal this ring. It does not matter if this seal is not perfect; it is merely to hold the coverslip in place. Return the preparation to the dessicator for a further day and then turn two layers of shellac varnish onto the coverslip to seal and finish it.

Most collections of small objects within a slide look far better presented when laid out on a grid rather than as a strewn slide. Suitable grids can be made either by reduction from a master on a photocopier, or by true photographic reduction. The former method using a photocopier tends to give a grey result, particularly if copying white on black. A photocopy reduction must also be turned through 90° at each successive reduction to prevent lateral distortion as the light sweeps the master copy. Darnton (1990) gives directions for making reduced grids directly onto film negative using line film, which can be developed in red safe light. The master is drawn with white ink onto black scraper board, and the letters added using rub-on transfers. A picture taken at 60 cm will give a 13 mm diameter circle, which can then be coated on the reverse with coloured car spray paint and glued into the cell. The best glue to use for this purpose is a glass bonding glue which is cured in the sun or by UV light.

5.8.2 Fluid mounts

Where possible specimens should be mounted in a resin mounting medium. This is not always possible: the tissue may not withstand fixing and hardening; the substrate or stain may be soluble in alcohol or be destroyed by the clearing medium. Stained preparations may be mounted in Farrants' or Apathy's medium, or a synthetic carboxymethyl cellulose mountant. These aqueous mountants are discussed in Chapter 7. Where larger, unstained specimens must be contained in a cell, a gelatin, glycerol jelly or an aqueous fluid mount is made. Any medium containing glycerol will tend to take up water on humid days and discharge it on dry days, and stained preparations cannot be mounted into glycerol jelly or glycerol mounts, since the dyes will leach out of the preparation.

Pure glycerol mounts are very difficult to seal, and should be avoided where gum media, glycerol jelly or aqueous preparations can be made. Aqueous fluid mounts can be used for most purposes where dehydration and clearing into a resin mount is not possible. The refractive index is low (ca. 1.3), and glycerol jelly should be used where the refractive index must be raised. Glycerol also provides a higher refractive index and is most suited for very delicate organisms that would otherwise collapse upon dehydration into either glycerol jelly, gelatin or gum media.

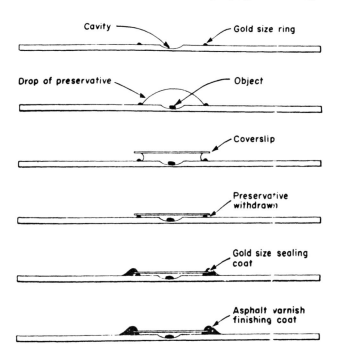

Figure 5.6: Preparation of a thin cavity or fluid mount. This method, illustrated using a cavity cell, is also the technique of choice when, alternatively, a thin cell is built up using successive rings turned on the slide. Where deeper cells are required, refer to *Figure 5.8*. Reproduced from Gray (1954).

The simplest fluid mounts of very small organisms can often be made using a cavity slide (*Figure 5.6*) in lieu of a cell. They are easier to seal against leaks, while the cavity keeps the organism central during preparation. For a very thin fluid mount, where an objective of high magnification is to be employed, turn a ring with Bioseal (NBS). A thicker ring can be built up successively with Clearseal (NBS) or gold-size; for large organisms use an aluminium ring to make the cell.

The cement ring should be about 0.4 mm smaller than the diameter of coverslip which is to be used. Similarly, the coverslip should be just larger than the internal, and just smaller than the external, diameter of the metal ring used to build the cell. If it is too small, then too large a gap has to be subsequently sealed with cement. If the ring is too large, and almost equivalent to the diameter of the coverslip, then sealing becomes impossible. Before cementing the ring onto the slide, check that the top and bottom surfaces are entirely flat; if any edge extrudes, rub it flat with fine emery paper, as for dry mounts.

Whether rings are turned on a slide, or are cemented on, they should be prepared a few days in advance to allow the gold-size, which hardens very slowly, to dry completely. The underside of the cell should be inspected in reflected light to ensure good adhesion. Where the glass slide acts as a mirror, and obscures the detail of the ring, adhesion has failed and the cell must be re-made, as it is liable to leak or let in microbes.

Where a thermoplastic cement is used to glue the ring to the slide, warm both prior to coating on a warming table (*Figure 5.7*), and coat the underside of the ring; remove any bubbles in the cement with a hot needle. Glue both slide and ring firmly together and move to a lower part of the table to cool gradually. The slide and ring should be weighted or clamped together while they cool off. Inspect the cell for good adhesion as before, and remove any internal exudate, first with a scalpel and then with a small

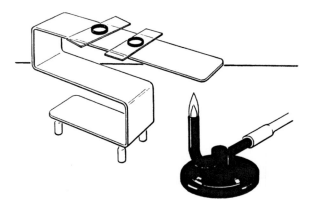

Figure 5.7:   The warming table. This may be constructed from a metre or so of alloy strip, with feet tapped into the base. A spirit lamp may equally well be used in place of the Bunsen burner. Reproduced from Gray (1954).

rag held in forceps and soaked in 1% potassium or sodium hydroxide. Take care, as concentrated alkalis will corrode aluminium rings. Wash the cell thoroughly, and dry off in a dessicator or warm cupboard.

Prior to filling the cell, turn a ring of gold-size onto the upper surface of the cell and allow this to dry over a maximum of 24 h to a rubbery consistency. If the ring is left too tacky, it may run into the mount. Any of the preservative fluids given can be used in these aqueous preparations. Formaldehyde is not ideal for invertebrates or single-celled plankton, but if it is used, it should be used unbuffered at 0.1%. Saturated camphor or chloroform water serve well for fresh-water Protozoa. Buffered or salt solutions should be avoided because they often throw down precipitates later. Any copper-containing fluids that have been used for fixing and preserving algal chloroplasts should be replaced with a colourless preservative, for example 2% formalin. The preservative should be boiled just before use to remove any dissolved air that would otherwise come out of solution in the finished preparation, and should be used immediately after cooling. Alternatively, the filled cell can be put in a dessicator under vacuum for a few hours to remove the air. Wipe the internal ring to the filled cell to dislodge any air bubbles that have become trapped when filling the cell with fluid.

Before applying the coverslip, ensure that the object is central in the cell, and that the preservative is in contact with the whole of the internal circumference of the cell to preclude air bubbles forming. Sufficient fluid should be applied to form a meniscus above the cell. Hold the coverslip between thumb and first finger and place it face down in the horizontal plane onto the meniscus of the fluid. This, together with just the right volume of preservative and not too dilute a sample, will help to prevent buoyant objects from being forced to the periphery of the cell. It is also a good idea to wait a little and allow the majority of the organisms to settle out before applying the coverslip. Draw out the excess fluid using a lint-free rag or segment of filter paper cut to an acute point.

Where the coverslip is to cover a large preparation, place it over most of the cell, as shown in the figure below, and push it on the last millimetre or so to coax out any air bubble that would otherwise become trapped at the upper edge of the cell (*Figure 5.8* has been exaggerated in this respect). The coverslip should not be lowered onto the preparation from one edge, nor dropped on: this will tend to displace the object. Once satisfactorily in position, push down the coverslip onto the gold-size ring with blunt forceps, and ensure a good seal all round.

Give the preparation a final wipe dry, and run a finishing layer of gold-size around the edge of the coverslip and the initial ring. Once this is dry, the preparation can be ringed twice with shellac varnish. Further details on preparing insect whole mounts and the use of glycerin jelly are given in Ives (1984).

Clearing and staining whole mount vertebrates. These techniques are beyond the scope of this monograph, and are generally used for

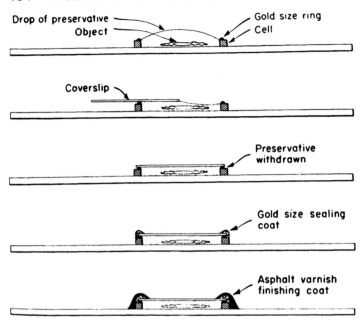

Figure 5.8:   Construction of a fluid mount in a cell. Reproduced from Gray (1954).

preparing anatomical museum specimens. The interested reader is referred to Dudzinski and Neff (1990) for a recent procedure.

5.9 Gum media

Gums are natural or synthetic. Apathy's and Farrants' media are of low
RI, while Berlèse's medium has chlorate hydrate added to it to raise the
RI. The lower RI renders the object opaque, while a higher medium is more
suited to viewing stained internal organs through the transparent integu-
ment. Gum media tend not to lend themselves well to deep cells nor indeed
to many small Protozoa or invertebrates, whose refractive indices equate
with the mounting medium with time, causing the object to 'vanish'.
However, it is a much simpler matter to mount hairs, scales and those
objects which do not behave so, than it is to mount them in a resinous
medium.

5.9.1 Glycerol jelly mounts

These solid gelatin-based mounts are a dispersion of gelatin in an amount
of glyerol calculated to give the appropriate RI. To prevent the jelly
cracking, which will occur if the specimen is mounted directly from water,

the organism must be infiltrated gradually with the glycerol via an alcohol–glycerol gradient. The alcohol both hardens and fixes the tissue, which otherwise might suffer from osmotic shock and diffusion currents during infiltration, and would certainly rot before the jelly stabilizes.

Ordinarily the object is brought to 95% alcohol, and then taken back to 70% alcohol, where sufficient glycerol is added to reduce the overall percentage of the glycerol to 50% after evaporation of the alcohol. The organism is then introduced into the molten jelly (kept at 10°C above its melting point) on a warm slide. The slide should be warm to reduce the rate at which the jelly sets; this prevents bubbles being trapped in the mount. Place a drop of mountant in the ring or cell on the slide. Add the organism via a Pasteur pipette. Truncate the tip with glasscutters and flame-polish the edges.

Fill the cell with molten jelly and displace any bubbles with a needle. Position the object with warmed, blunt-ended forceps or a seeker. Remove the slide from the warming table and let the object settle onto the slide and the jelly solidify, leaving a dome slightly raised above the level of the cell. The coverslip is taken and smeared with 50% glycerol (or breathed on), and pressed gently into place with the warmed press shown in *Figure 5.9*. By this means, the top layer of glycerol jelly melts and seals the coverslip into place while leaving the object undisturbed. Weight down the coverslip and leave the entire preparation in a warm place or on the coolest part of the hot-plate to cool gradually to room temperature and allow the osmotic forces to equilibrate. Once the preparation is at room

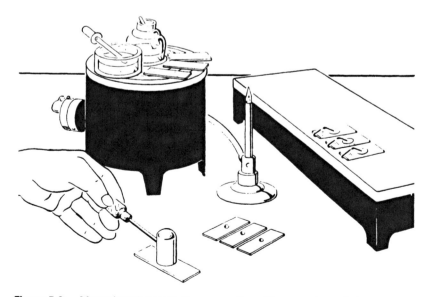

Figure 5.9:   Mounting glycerol jelly preparations. The press is made from 20 mm diameter aluminium rod, faced-off flat at one end. A 50 mm length of 3–4 mm brass tube is tapped into the rod, and terminated with an insulating wooden handle. Three slides, with the paper-clip weights described in *Figure 7.1*, can be seen in the background. Reproduced from Gray (1954).

temperature it can be placed in the fridge to set any extraneous jelly, which can then be trimmed away.

The cell is finished by first wiping away any excess jelly. Any remaining glycerol is likewise removed with another rag soaked in 95% ethanol. A sealing ring of Reuter's gelatin-dichromate cement (Gray, 1954) is applied, and allowed to dry thoroughly.

Reuter's gelatin-dichromate cement

Gelatin	20 g
Potassium dichromate	0.5 g
Distilled water	100 ml

Dissolve the gelatin in 90 ml of water, cool, and add the potassium dichromate dissolved in the remaining water. An alternative formula calls for the water to be saturated with oil of thyme, and to soak the gelatin overnight before melting and adding 10 ml of 5% potassium dichromate.

The whole preparation is wiped again with a cloth soaked in 95% ethanol, and a second sealing ring applied. Once this has also been allowed to dry, and the preparation wiped again a third time, a ring of gold-size is applied, followed by two of shellac or enamel. If the preparations crack due to an insufficient amount of glycerol, tap the coverslip sharply to break it, remove the specimen in a jelly block and soak in 50% glycerol in ethanol for 1–2 weeks. Consider the specimen as fresh, and remount.

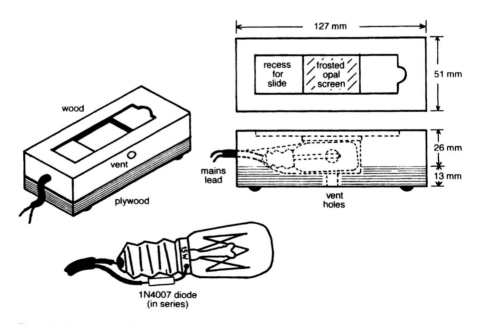

Figure 5.10: A warming box for glycerol jelly mounts. The suggested illuminant is a 240 V 15 W refrigerator bulb, with a 1N4007 diode in series to reduce the voltage, and thus the heat output. Ventilation holes are drilled in the bottom and side of the plywood carcase. The reduced light permits easy use of the box under a stereo-microscope. For the glycerol jelly protocol, see *Section 7.2*. Reproduced with permission from Mr Brian Adams.

A description of a portable heating box for mounting in glycerol jelly has been constructed by Brian Adams, and I am grateful for his permission to reproduce this (*Figure 5.10*). The carcase is made of plywood as indicated; the incorporation of a car lamp as a heating element means that the equipment can be used in the field. A thin film of gelatin-agar cast onto a microscope slide can be used to culture microbes for examination (Robinow, 1975). The medium around the inoculated area can be sufficiently reduced in size to fit under a coverslip and be temporarily sealed.

5.9.2 Glycerol fluid mounts

Because of the difficulty of sealing glycerol mounts, cells built up of cement rings turned on the slide are preferable to those of aluminium. The object is brought into glycerol through an ethanol gradient. Use absolute alcohol, dried over a molecular sieve, to prevent altering the RI by dilution of the glycerol with any traces of water. The glycerol should be added gradually, 1 ml at a time, over 24 h, to about a 20% concentration. The ethanol is then allowed to evaporate away, leaving the object in pure glycerol, from where it can be transferred to fresh glycerol for mounting.

Some whole mounts of crustaceans and insect larvae can be rendered transparent by gradually replacing the infiltrated preservative with glycerol: a 60% volume of glycerol should be run under a 40% volume of the preservative in a small vial. If organisms are dropped in, they will rest on the phase layer. Shake the bottle daily (if the organism is sufficiently robust) until all the fluid is mixed, then mount the organisms from this mixture as a glycerol mount.

A glycerol-filled cell can be sealed using molten gelatin, or Reuter's gelatin-dichromate cement referred to above. The coverslip is held in place by the cement whilst cleaning up and ringing the preparation. All traces of glycerol must be entirely removed with alcohol, as described above for glycerol jelly mounts, before ringing with gold-size and varnish or enamel. An illustrated method for sealing glycerol mounts under straight-edged coverslips has been published by Gray (1954).

References

Abele JS, Miller TR, King EB. (1985) Smearing techniques for the concentration of particles from fine needle aspiration biopsy. *Diagnost. Cytopathol.* **1**, 59–65.

Balasubramanian A. (1979) Improved imprinting technique for study of plant tissues. *Stain Technol.* **54**, 177–180.

Bentley SA, Marshall PN, Trobaugh FE. (1980) Standardization of the Romanowsky-staining procedure: an overview. *Anal. Quant. Cytol.* **2**, 15–18.

Boon ME, Drijver JS. (1985) *Routine Cytological Staining Techniques: Theoretical Background and Practice.* Macmillan Press Ltd, Basingstoke.

Bradbury S. (1973) *Peacock's Elementary Microtechnique,* 4th revised edn. Edward Arnold, London.

Brocklehurst K. (1993) An introduction to displaying and counting chromosomes. *Quekett J. Microsc.* **37**, 56–63.

Cobb N, Slater BN, Beck S. (1990) A new filter technique permitting traditional histopathological assessment of fine needle aspiration specimens. *Med. Lab. Sci.* **47**, 172–181.

Coleman DV, Chapman PA. (eds) (1989) *Clinical Cytotechnology.* Butterworths, London.

Collins CH, Lyne PM, Grange JM. (1989) *Collins and Lyne's Microbiological Methods,* 6th edn. Butterworths, London.

Costa M, Buffa R, Furness JB, Solcia E. (1980) Immunohistochemical localization of polypeptides in peripheral autonomic nerves using whole mount preparations. *Histochemistry* **65**, 157–165.

Darnton B. (1990) The collection and mounting of recent Foraminifera. *Microsc. Bull.* (of the Quekett Microscopical Club) **16**, 14–17.

Dick DAT. (1955) An easily made tissue culture perfusion chamber. *Q. J. Microscop. Sci.* **96**, 363–369.

van Driel-Kulker AMJ, Mesher WE, van der Burg MJM, Ploem JS. (1987) Preparation of cells from paraffin-embedded tissue for cytometry and cytomorphologic evaluation. *Anal. Quant. Cytol. Histol.* **9**, 225–231.

Duarte LA. (1991) A new technique for facilitating studies of scant cell specimens. *Biotechnic Histochem.* **66**, 200–202.

Dudzinski KM, Neff NA. (1990) A technique for the combination of clearing, staining, and injecting small mammals. *Stain Technol.* **65**, 113–118.

Gray B. (1964) Sputum cytodiagnosis in bronchial carcinoma: a comparative study of two methods. *Lancet* **ii**, 549.

Gray P. (1954) *The Microtomist's Formulary and Guide.* Blakiston, New York.

Gray P. (1964) *Handbook of Basic Microtechnique,* 3rd edn. McGraw-Hill, New York.

Guyer M. (1953) *Animal Micrology,* 5th revised edn. University of Chicago Press, Chicago.

Humason GL. (1972) *Animal Tissue Techniques,* 3rd edn. WH Freeman, San Francisco, CA.

Ives E. (1984) Whole mounts of insects. *Microscopy* **35**, 45–51.

Kok LP, Boon ME, Ouwerkerk-Noordam E, Gerrits PO. (1986) The application of a microwave technique for the preparation of cell blocks from sputum. *J. Microsc.* **144**, 193–199.

Kung ITM, Long BFC, Chan JKC. (1989) Rehydration of air dried smears: application in body cavity fluid cytology. *J. Clin. Pathol.* **42**,113.

Lee TK. (1982) The value of imprint cytology in tumor diagnosis. A retrospective study of 522 cases in northern China. *Acta Cytol.* **26**, 169–171.

Marson JE. (1983) *Practical Microscopy.* Northern Biological Supplies, Ipswich.

Orell SR, Sterrett GF, Walters MN-J, Whitaker D. (1992) *Manual and Atlas of Fine Needle Aspiration Cytology,* 2nd edn. Churchill Livingstone, Edinburgh.

Pentz S, Hörler H. (1992) A variable cell culture chamber for 'open' and 'closed' cultivation, perfusion and high microscopic resolution of living cells. *J. Microsc.* **167**, 97–103.

Robinow CF. (1975) The preparation of yeasts for light microscopy. *Methods Cell Biol.* **11**, 1–22.

Sevcik G, Guttenberger H, Grill D. (1993) A perfusion chamber with temperature regulation. *Biotechnic Histochem.* **68**, 229–236.

Sumner AT. (1989) Chromosome banding. In *Light Microscopy in Biology* (ed. AJ Lacey). IRL Press, Oxford, pp. 279–314.

Tribe CR. (1965) Cytological diagnosis of breast tumours by the imprint method. *J. Clin. Pathol.* **18**, 1–39.

Wagstaffe R, Fidler JH. (1955,1968) *Preservation of Natural History Specimens,* Vols I and II. Witherby, London.

6 Staining and Dyeing

The visibility of the tissue is commonly increased by using compounds which differentially absorb visible light to produce a coloured preparation. Dyes absorb light; a dye appears red because it absorbs all the colours of the spectrum except red light, which is allowed to pass.

To study internal structural elements (rather than merely to introduce contrast for studying external features) the stain(s) must act selectively so that specific features of the preparation can be studied alongside differently coloured tissues. The most effective results arise from using a basic and acid stain, preferably of complementary colours, in succession. The basic stains, which are generally used for chromatin, are chosen from the ends of the visible spectrum, while the background counter-stains are chosen from the more central region. This is because the eye perceives yellow and green-yellow hues as unsaturated; if small inclusions and organelles (e.g. chromosomes) were to be stained thus, they would effectively disappear against the more highly saturated red or blue background.

6.1 Nomenclature

The term 'staining' is generally used to include all methods of colouring tissue. Baker (1958) distinguishes between dyeing and staining; the former process involves the tissue taking up only the dye molecule from solution, leaving the solvent. In the latter case both dye solute and solvent are taken up. The simplest distinction between staining and dyeing is that defined by Kiernan (1990) and Boon and Drijver (1985): where colouring is caused by linking a dye molecule and tissue substrate, the process is called dyeing; if the tissue is stained by solution contact alone, the process is called staining. In this book, the term 'staining' will be used throughout to avoid confusion. For a complete discussion of the mechanisms of staining and dyeing see Kiernan (1990) and Boon and Drijver (1985). For a more advanced treatise, see Horobin (1982, 1988).

The chromophore contains the coloured part of the stain molecule, which is usually an aromatic resonance hybrid. Since aromatic compounds rarely ionize, an ionic component is required within the molecule to allow

159

reaction with tissue sites. The auxochrome is the ionizing part of the stain that ligates, or attaches, to the tissue, often enhancing the intensity of the stain in the process. In empirical methods, the dye–tissue attachment is mostly incompletely understood. Where the exact localization of dye within tissue is known, which is rare, the method is known as a histochemical one and can be used as a precise analytical technique.

Stains are classified according to their chromophores, although their visible action may be modified by a small group of recurrent auxochromes For example, Eosin Y and Erythrosine B differ only in their auxochromes: eosin possesses bromine, and erythrosine iodine. The latter stain absorbs more of the longer, red wavelengths, and is bluer than eosin.

There is no single logical system of nomenclature; for instance light green may be the acid dye light green SF yellowish, or either of the two very different basic dyes methyl green or malachite green. These three dyes have all been sold in the past under the generic label Light Green. The dye Congo red is so named not because it came from Africa, but solely because it appeared on the market when the Congo became an independent state.

6.2 Staining action

Many dyes attach to ionic radicals within the tissue, and are very much pH dependent. Nuclei $(PO_4)^{2-}$, mucus and cartilage $(SO_3)^-$, and some proteins $(COO)^-$ have acidic amino acid residues in their structure capable of interacting with basic, cationic dyes. They are therefore referred to as basiphilic. Alternatively, erythrocytes and some leucocytes have free NH_2^+ groups, are basic in nature and can combine with acidic, anionic dyes. These tissues are acidophilic. The terms 'basiphil' and 'acidophil' refer to the groups of the tissue which react with the dye, and not to the pH of the intracellular fluid.

Amphoteric dyes behave as alkaline dyes in acidic solutions and vice versa. This is due to a supression of ionized acidic groups of the dye in acid solution, leaving an *excess* of ionized basic groups. Thus, a basic dye can be used at a pH on the acidic side of its iso-electric point (e.g. basic fuchsin in the Ziehl-Neelsen method). The isoelectric point is the pH where the acid and basic groups balance each other out giving rise to a neutral salt. Most unmordanted basic (cationic) stains are very soluble in water, and must be dehydrated rapidly. This is less critical for acid stains (e.g. eosin), but both these stains must usually be mounted in resinous media to avoid diffusion and fading from the target site.

Generally, dyes used to stain the chromatin are basic, and those used to stain the cytoplasm acidic. An 'exception' is the stain Bismark brown, which was originally included in the cytoplasmic component of

Papanicolaou's original formula, but is now often omitted since it plays no significant part in staining cytoplasm. Non-ionic stains (e.g. fat 'stains') soluble in dehydrating and transition media must be mounted in aqueous mountants. The dyes which impart colour to lipids are not truly stains, but lysochromes, which act by phase-partitioning of the dye preferentially into the lipid from the solvent (e.g. Oil red 0, Sudan black B, Nile blue A). Full dicussion of the mechanistic concepts of staining can be found in Horobin (1988, 1990) and Horobin *et al.* (1990).

The fixative used in the protocol can influence the staining reaction of the tissue. Unfixed tissue takes up little stain, but fixatives unmask ionic groups and enhance staining. Formalin fixation initially favours acid dyes, inducing basiphilia, but overfixation with formalin will impair nuclear staining by haematoxylin. Other fixatives (e.g. dichromate) increase tissue acidophilia, and cause greater staining avidity.

6.2.1 Mordants

A mordant links a dye to the tissue, forming a combination termed a 'lake'. Regardless of the nature of the charge on the original dye, the lake is invariably basic in action. Haematoxylin must be mordanted to the tissue by a metal ion in order to stain effectively as dye–mordant–tissue lake (*Figure 6.1*). This is because the dye is amphoteric, and because of opposing charges on its molecule would not bind sufficiently strongly to the tissue. Staining by haematoxylin is therefore indirect, whereas non-amphoteric dyes can be applied directly.

Separate dye-baths may be employed with indirect dyes to allow greater control of staining, although the dye and mordant are usually combined in the case of haematoxylin. Aluminium is usually the mordant of choice,

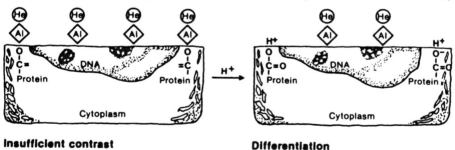

Insufficient contrast   **Differentiation**

He Haematein

Al Metal ion

Figure 6.1: The mechanism of mordanting and differentiation. The mordant (here the positively charged hydrated aluminium ion chelate is shown) increases the affinity of (the negatively charged) haematoxylin for the electron-donor groups of the tissue substrate sites. The illustration shows the phosphate groups of nucleic acids and carboxyl groups of proteins forming lakes. By differentiation, hydrogen ions selectively replace the weaker carboxyl lake. Lengthy immersion in acid will over-differentiate, removing the haematoxylin from the nucleic acid (illustration courtesy of Merck).

added directly to the haematoxylin as an alum salt. Iron is the other common metal mordant; the ferric ions also act as a powerful oxidant, obviating the need for sodium iodate. While iron haematoxylins are ready for immediate use, they have a negligible lifetime of a few hours, and take much longer to stain tissue, although a much wider range of tissue structures are demonstrated. Accentuators, which may also be called accelerators in the neurological literature, increase the avidity of a tissue for a dye without acting as a mordant or forming a lake.

Besides dyeing, other methods of colouring tissue are by metallic impregnation (in electron microscopy, silver or immunogold methods), by trapping (e.g. the Gram reaction), by preferential solution within the cell without attachment to any cell component (lysochromes), or by displacement (Clark, 1979) which occurs when a solution of one dye is used to replace another, the most common example being the phloxine-tartrazine stain for cellular inclusions. Negative staining of the background, against which the bacterial capsule can be seen, is another type chiefly used for micro-organisms. Vital stains (Section 6.8) may be taken up by phagocytosis, in contrast to the more common diffusion of the dye molecule into the tissue. Another widely used method of staining results from the uptake and conversion of colourless compounds (leuco-bases) to a coloured reaction product by the cell. This last category includes many enzymatic and immunological histochemical methods. Some chromophoric groups with double bonds may be reduced in the presence of hydrogen to form saturated, colourless compounds or leuco-dyes, which may be re-oxidized to their former states. A leuco-base is reduced not by hydrogen, but by hydroxyl ions.

6.2.2 Metachromasia

Unlike leuco-compounds, a dye which can change its colour without a change in its chemical structure is said to be metachromatic. This is due to the molecular stacking of the dye molecules, and the phenomenon is influenced by changes in water content, concentration and solvent, pH and temperature. A metachromatic dye can be simply tested by dissolving the dye in water at a low concentration. Increasing the amount of dye will result in a colour change, which is reversible upon dilution. Most metachromatic dyes are thiazines (thionin, toluidine blue, Azure A and B), but eosin, methyl violet, acridine orange, safranin, Alcian blue 8GX and Congo red are also included.

The monomeric forms of the thiazine dyes are blue (orthochromatic), changing through purple to red with increasing dye concentration, pH, decreasing temperature and polar (water) solvency. Adding salts to the staining solution increases metachromasia, while polar molecules such as alcohols retard the effect. Tissues with high charge densities and hydrated tissues particularly favour metachromasia, which can, in some cases, disappear on dehydration of the tissue (in organic solvents) during the course of preparation. The best example of metachromasia is the staining of blood films with the R-G stain (Section 6.6.1), and hydrated tissues such as mucopolysaccharides.

6.3 Nuclear stains

The most widely used nuclear stain is the natural dye haematoxylin extracted from the red heartwood of the leguminous tree *Haematoxylon campechianum*. Carmine stains are derived from the fat bodies of the female scale insect *Dactylopius cacti*. For further details see Baker (1958), and for a history of staining, Clark and Kasten (1973).

6.3.1 Haematoxylin

Haematoxylin is colourless, and the dyeing action is due to the oxidation product haematein. Haematein is not the same as haematin, which is the oxygen-carrying moiety of haemoglobin. Oxidation (ripening) of hae-matoxylin to the active dye takes place either by artificial means or natural sunlight. Since the further oxidation products of haematein (oxy-hae-matein and haematoxylic acid) are useless for dyeing, these nuclear dyes have a limited shelf-life. While chemically ripened haematoxylins are ready for immediate use, those formulae which call for slower natural ripening by sunlight are often stable for years rather than weeks or months. The shelf-life of all haematoxylin mixtures can be prolonged by storage in amber bottles filled to the brim, to exclude air, in the dark.

Sodium iodate is normally used for chemical ripening. Baker and Jordan (1953) have published a series of modified formulae which are half-oxidized. During use in the staining baths, a metallic scum of hae-matein and further oxidation products of the dye will collect on the surface. The dye must therefore be filtered daily, or before use. Exhaustion of the haematoxylin is seen when the nuclei no longer stain crisply, and the overall effect on the section is a muddy blue-grey, rather than crisp, well-differentiated detail.

Staining is usually regressive. That is, overstaining is carried out followed by differentiation (under microscopical control) in dilute acid or excess mordant. This is not always easy to accomplish, and where the mordant ferric ammonium sulphate is used as a differentiator, over-oxi-dation of the haematoxylin may leave a yellow tinge to the cytoplasm. This either impairs contrast for the reasons explained above, or interferes with subsequent counter-staining.

Alum haematoxylins are simpler and quicker to use, but are very sensitive to any subsequent acid stain, which differentiates them from the tissue. Iron haematoxylins are acid-fast and give black nuclei, which is useful for photomicrography. It is possible to confer acid-fastness upon alum haematoxylins by using them in conjunction with celestine blue to stain nuclei. The subtler staining and speedier result are retained; this method is given in Section 6.5.1. For this reason, and also for ease of use by those beginning in microtechnique, two long-lived progressive stains have been developed and published by Baker (1964) and Gill *et al.* (1974). Both these stains are given below. Further details of haematoxylins and mordants can be found in Stevens (1990).

Baker's Haematal 8
Equal volumes of the following two solutions are mixed. Both the stock solutions and the working solution are stable.

Aluminium sulphate (0.025 M) ($Al_2(SO_4)_3.16H_2O$)	1.576 g
Distilled water, to make up to	1000 ml
Haematein (0.00625 M)	0.188 g
Ethylene glycol (ethanediol), 50% (aq) v/v	100 ml

Where Zenker's fixative is used, restrict the duration of fixation to 6 h. Good staining of sections is achieved in 2–15 min. Excess stain is washed off with a wash bottle of distilled water—no blueing is necessary. This stain will not overstain, whole mounts may be stained in it: immerse organisms for several hours. Wash away excess stain using 0.0125 M aluminium sulphate, followed by a thorough water wash.

Gill's haematoxylin

Distilled water	730 ml
Ethylene glycol	250 ml
Haematoxylin	2 g
Sodium iodate	0.2 g
Aluminium sulphate ($Al_2(SO_4)_3.18H_2O$)	17.6 g
Acetic acid (glacial)	20 ml
(or citric acid	1 g)

Mix in the order given in a flask, using a magnetic stirrer, for 1 h at room temperature. The stain can be used immediately.

Celestine blue

Celestine blue B or R	10 g
5% ferric ammonium sulphate	860 ml
Glycerol	140 ml
Sulphuric acid (conc.)	5 ml

Use only the clear violet crystals of ferric alum, dissolve them in cold water with stirring. Grind the celestine blue to a paste with the sulphuric acid—*care!* Gradually add the saturated alum and mix well. Add the glycerol, place in an oven at 56°C overnight to dissolve. Cool and filter through double sheets of filter paper. This stain can be used to mordant alum haematoxylins, allowing counterstaining with an acid stain, such as van Gieson.

Some workers add 4% triacetin (1,2,3,-triacetylglycerol) to the dehydrating alcohols on the tissue processor. This not only enhances nuclear staining, but also improves the microtomy of dense tissues.

6.3.2 Differentiation

Where the alum nuclear stain needs to be differentiated, use 1% acid in 70% ethanol. The most commonly used acid is hydrochloric, but nitric and acetic acid are sometimes called for. Iron haematoxylins use a dilute mordant solution (e.g. 5% ferric ammonium sulphate). Methods staining with cresyl violet use clove oil, an essential transition medium, for differentiation, although 1% acetic acid can be used, since this is the solvent for cresyl violet. Other stains may be differentiated on a similar basis, using an excess of the dye solvent.

6.3.3 'Blueing'

In most regions the tap water is sufficiently alkaline to be able to impart a good blue colour to the nuclei in 2–5 min, but where this is not achieved, or where artificial blueing is preferred for standardization, use Scott's tap water substitute, or 0.1% sodium bicarbonate. Both solutions are at about pH 8.1. Scott's tap water substitute may be stored for many months, but should be filtered before use.

Scott's tap water substitute

Sodium bicarbonate	3.5 g
Magnesium sulphate	20 g
Tap water, to make up to	1000 ml
Thymol preservative	A small crystal

Where material has been fixed in an acid fixative, or one that requires copious washing before deydrating and embedding, it is essential that this step be carried out *very* rigorously to avoid there being any acid left in the tissue at the commencement of staining (Section 2.10). This can interfere with the initial intensity of stain and its distribution, and can promote fading (particularly of the azure blue dyes) on storage. Where washing after blueing is omitted, or is insufficient, a milky film is seen on the underside of the slide, and small refractile particles may be seen in the preparation.

6.3.4 Other nuclear stains

Since haematoxylin is the most ubiquitous nuclear stain and is fast in both aqueous and organic solvents, there is rarely any requirement for an alternative nuclear stain except when supplies of the natural dye are threatened. Digoxygenin, a histochemical substrate often conjugated to nucleic acids and used as an *in situ* hybridization probe, is a dark blue-black colour (like Heidenhain's haematoxylin) and is alcohol-soluble. Using methyl green as a counterstain tends to promote leaching of the stain into the aqueous mountant. Ideally, for photography the counterstain should be of the complementary colour to the blue of digoxygenin—i.e. red. This may be achieved in one of two ways. Either the tissue may be stained directly with Kernechtrot (nuclear fast red, calcium red, CI 60760) for 5–10 min and mounted directly from water, or else a 1% solution of nuclear fast red may be precipitated *in situ* using 5% phosphotungstic or 1% phosphomolybdic acid. The direct method gives a low contrast burgundy red, while the precipitation method gives a scarlet result of higher contrast.

6.3.5 Carmine

Historically, the use of carmine preceded that of haematoxylin. It is now used primarily as a whole mount stain, rather than for nuclei, although the latter role is still useful where the counterstain is to be in green, rather than red or orange. The active component of the staining mixture is carminic acid, although the less pure carmine dye is used to make up the stain.

6.3.6 Safranin

This natural dye is largely used for plant tissues, and is usually employed as a 1% stain of Safranin O in water, 50% ethyl alcohol or 100% 2-ethoxy ethanol. It can also be used for wood staining as a ripe, saturated solution in 50% ethanol in 3% aqueous aniline. The quality of this natural dye varies much more between batches than either haematoxylin or carmine.

6.3.7 Synthetic nuclear dyes

Celestine blue has already been mentioned, as suitable for use in conjuction with alum haematoxylins. In the early 1970s a worldwide haematoxylin shortage led to a search for man-made substitutes (Lillie *et al.*, 1975). Other synthetic dyes that have been advocated are Chromoxine Cyanine R, Tetracycline and Fluorone black.

6.4 Counterstains

These are mostly anionic stains, which colour the cytoplasm of the cell. Counterstains are used to give contrast to the major dye component in the preparation. They should be pale to avoid masking the specific stain, should not remove it, nor require differentiation which would do so. Since most counterstains are direct and do not require a mordant, no differentiation is needed. Staining is therefore controlled progressively.

6.4.1 Eosin

This xanthene dye is commonly used as a 0.1–0.5% aqueous solution. It is best diluted from a 5% stock solution, to which a few crystals of thymol or a few drops of 10% formalin have been added to inhibit mould growth. Thymol is to be preferred to phenol, which can leach out nuclear stains with time, and cause fading. Even where mould growth has occurred, good staining can be secured by filtering the dye. Eosin filters very slowly: allow 1 h to fill a 300 ml staining bath, so that work is not held up!

Excess dye can be removed from the section with a brief water wash, or differentiation in 70% alcohol without disturbing the haematoxylin nuclear stain. Eosin fluoresces yellow-green, and its staining intensity is pH and solvent dependent, increasing in alcohol and with pH. Fixatives containing mercuric and dichromate ions render tissue more avid for eosin, as does 0.05% acetic acid; 1% calcium chloride is a good mordant. Eosin Y WS is the most common eosin dye; two lesser used stains are Erythrosin B, 0.5% in 95% alcohol; Phloxine B, 0.5% aqueous with a few drops of acetic acid. Phloxine, 1% in 90% alcohol or 0.5% aqueous, and Biebrich scarlet WS, 0.1% aqueous have also been advocated, but these are not as amenable to differentiation as eosin. Which counterstain is selected largely depends upon personal preference.

6.4.2 Other counterstains

Although H & E is the most commonly used oversight stain in animal histology, van Gieson's is also employed to demonstrate connective tissue, and other fields use slightly different protocols. In cytology the Papanicolaou stain, employing Eosin-Orange G is ubiquitous, and botanists generally use Fast green FCF as a counterstain for safranin. The reader is referred to Gray (1954), Bradbury (1973) and Clark (1981) for other protocols.

6.5 General staining procedures

The area chosen for staining work should be well lit by top lighting, and face preferably onto windows. There should be at least one sink with two cold water taps. Where it is possible to install a piped supply of distilled water, this is better than having containers (5 l minimum) which need refilling. There should, in any case, be an adequate supply of distilled water for making up stains and for washing tissues as required. Where stains are made up in alcohol this should be absolute ethanol unless otherwise stated.

Stock reagents and stains should be kept in a cupboard at floor level in clearly marked bottles. Flammable reagents should be kept in a flameproof cupboard, and both cupboards should be kept locked when not in routine use. Stoppered bottles are best, since screw-top bottles tend to promote the formation of crystalline deposits of stain around the screw, which can lead to contamination. Use amber bottles for silver staining reagents and others which require protection from the light. Work surfaces are best covered with a disposable absorbent sheet such as Benchkote Plus (Whatman).

Those reagents which are used frequently can be kept in designated dropper or wash bottles and Coplin jars. Stains in Coplin jars and staining baths are prone to oxidation, even with a lid, and will require filtering, perhaps on a daily basis. Suitable glass or plastic must be used where a protocol calls for stains to be heated or microwaved.

The use of heat for staining, like fixation, is best avoided; where this is necessary to reduce the time involved it is best done using microwaves. Where stains are heated without microwaving, it is best to use a water-bath, and pour the hot stain onto the slide to stain the tissue. Heating the slide directly by means of a naked flame with the stain on top of the slide, or boiling the stain in a test-tube, is not advised as many stains are volatile and made up in flammable diluents.

A basic bench microscope is required for checking the progress of the staining microscopically. It is best to have a fixed, rather than a mechanical, stage as the former is easier to keep clean. A 4:1, 10:1 and 25:1 battery of achromat objectives will serve for this instrument. When checking the progress of staining, a coverglass should be dropped on with water to form a temporary mount. The coverglass should be eased off carefully by swinging it off the plane of the slide, rather than by picking it up at one edge, as this will not damage the tisssue section. Where there is a risk of damage, merely examine the section quickly without the use of a cover-glass. The use of a coverglass allows a more leisurely examination of the preparation without it drying out. A water-immersion objective would obviate the need for a coverslip, but these tend to give a high magnification of a small field of view, which is not what is required whilst assessing the progress of staining.

Staining baths should be laid out near the sink in a manner that allows the work to progress without crossing over baths holding other reagents (*Figure 6.2*). Dripping can cause contamination, and interrupting the flow of work can lead to error. When a stain is poured out, it should be done so that the label is not masked by any drips.

Slides are dewaxed in xylene or toluene where necessary, and any pigment removed before staining (Section 6.10). Once in water, the sections should not be allowed to dry until they have been mounted from the transition medium and a coverslip sealed in place. Further details on the

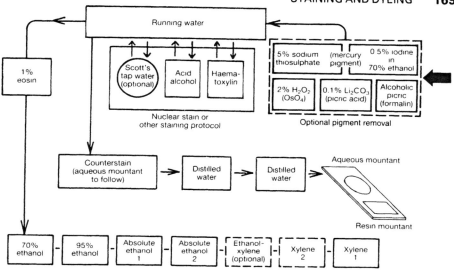

Figure 6.2:   The sequence of staining, dehydration and transition baths.

Table 6.1:   Points to watch when staining

Do	Don't
Make up stains with good quality reagents and distilled water	Direct jets of wash water at the section
Filter stains made from stock powders unless directed otherwise	Cut short the staining times
Flood the slide well	Allow water stains or volatile reagents to evaporate off leaving the sections dry
Rinse the slides well front and back	Dehydrate too rapidly, unless directed otherwise
Use a good mounting medium	Store specimens in sunlight where stains will rapidly fade

removal of the embedding medium prior to staining, dehydration are given in Chapter 3 and mounting in Chapter 7. Celloidin sections are floated through the reagents, and attached to the slide only after they have been stained. They require longer staining times, and mounting is more difficult in that the edges of the section tend to wrinkle and can trap air bubbles. An intermediate bath of carbol-xylene is used to clear the sections, as they do not clear in xylene alone; the sections are flooded and blotted twice in xylene to remove the phenol before mounting.

To conclude, histological processing and staining is as much an art as it is a science. There are some 'dos' and 'don'ts' which apply to histological technique in general, and staining in particular, that are set out in *Table 6.1*.

6.5.1 Selected staining protocols

H & E

1.	Stain sections in haematoxylin.	10 min
2.	Wash in running tap water.	
3.	Differentiate in 1% HCl in 70% ethanol.	2–3 dips
4.	Blue in Scott's tap water.	
5.	Wash in tap water.	
6.	Stain sections in eosin.	30–60 sec
7.	Wash briefly in tap water.	
8.	Dehydrate, starting with 70% ethanol, via 80% and 95% to two changes of absolute ethanol.	30–60 sec each
9.	Transfer through two changes of xylene and mount in DPX.	

Results

Nuclei	Purple, blue or black, depending upon the haematoxylin and extent of differentiation
Basiphil cytoplasm Cartilage }	Purple
Cytoplasm and collagen	Pink
Muscle fibres	Red
Erythrocytes Eosinophil granules }	Scarlet red

The success of the classic H & E stain depends upon correct differentiation of the eosin, which is metachromatic. Both the quick water rinse and lower (70%) alcohols will extract the stain. Sufficient should be removed to give the results above. Calcium chloride (1%) can be added to the haematoxylin to increase avidity of the eosin, which is the less fast of the two dyes—if it remains too densely bound to the tissues during dehydration, add a few drops of ammonia solution to the 70% alcohol.

Haematoxylin and van Gieson

1.	Stain with alum haematoxylin	5 min
	or iron haematoxylin (e.g. Weigert's).	25 min
2.	Wash in running tap water.	
3.	Differentiate in 1% HCl in 70% ethanol.	2–3 dips
4.	Blue in Scott's tap water.	
5.	Wash in tap water.	
6.	Stain in celestine blue (if alum haematoxylin is used).	5 min
7.	Wash in running tap water.	
8.	Stain in van Gieson's solution.	5 min
9.	Dehydrate quickly.	
10.	Pass through transition medium and mount.	

Results

Cell nuclei	Dark brown/black

Collagen	Bright red
Muscle	Brown or yellow
Elastic tissue	Blue-black
Erythrocytes	Yellow

Dehydrate fairly quickly through the lower alcohols, without washing, to retain the van Gieson stain. With this method an iron haematoxylin must be used, or the alum haematoxylin mordanted using celestine blue, because the picric acid in van Gieson's stain will leach out the nuclear stain.

Baker's Haematal 8 and Biebrich scarlet
1. The sections are stained with Haematal 8.   12–15 min
2. Wash 0.0125 M aluminium sulphate followed by
    a thorough wash in water.
3. Stain with 0.1% Biebrich scarlet WS.   2–5 min
4. Wash briefly in water.
5. Dehydrate, clear and mount in a resinous mountant.

6.5.2 Stains for glycerol jelly mounts

Many stains fade when mounted in glycerol jelly. Brat's and du Jardin's methods (Snoek, 1983) are claimed to be very useful, in particular for plant sections, for retarding fading. These methods are suited to slide-mounted sections supported on a staining rack, but free-floating sections may equally well be stained with a slight modification of the protocol. Du Jardin's method is suitable for resinous mountants.

Brat's method

Astrablue	0.25 g
Tartaric acid	1.0 g
Distilled water to	100 ml
Basic fuchsin	0.5 g
96% ethanol	100 ml
Concentrated ammonia solution	10 ml

Add the concentrated ammonia to the alcoholic basic fuchsin solution until it becomes colourless.

Protocol
1. Bring the sections to distilled water for staining.
2. Replace the water by drops of ammonical fuchsin.   5 min
3. Rinse in distilled water, until a red colour is seen.
4. Counterstain with 0.25% Astrablue.   30 sec
5. Rinse in distilled water.   1 min
6. Immerse or float sections in 30% (aq) glycerol jelly.   20 min
7. Immerse or float sections in 50% (aq) glycerol jelly.   20 min
8. Immerse or float sections in 70% (aq) glycerol jelly.   20 min
8. Immerse or float sections in 90% (aq) glycerol jelly.   20 min
9. Mount in glycerol jelly and seal (Section 5.9.1).

Results

Nuclei	Blue
Cellulose	Bright-blue
Lignified tissue	Purple-red

A gradual replacement of glycerol for water avoids cracking of the set mountant; whole mounts are usually made from an alcohol–glycerol mixture.

6.5.3 Stains for resin-embedded material

As stated in Chapter 3, paraffin wax-embedded tissues accept a much wider range of different stains. Nevertheless, the advantages of using resin-embedded tissues for microscopy are such that many methods for staining resin sections have been published. For a review of stains suitable for semi-thin resin sections, see Hayat (1975). Another, more recent, review has also been published (Scala *et al.*, 1993) of staining techniques for resin sections. In addition, Scala and his colleagues report the sequential use of common dyes to give a vivid polychrome stain for acrylic resin. The stains given below are the most commonly used; Stevenel's stain, whilst not given here, is reported as particularly good for high resolution microscopy on plastic sections (del Cerro *et al.*, 1980).

Toluidine blue
Stain the section with 1% toluidine blue in 1% acetic acid. The stain can be applied regressively and differentiated with 0.1% acetic acid, but progressive staining can often give a better result. Times vary, but start with 20 sec.

Richardson's stain
This is a general oversight stain for resin sections. Mix together equal volumes of the following and double-filter.

1% Azure II in distilled water.
1% methylene blue in 1% borax.

To stain semi-thin sections, drop the stain onto dried sections on a hot-plate at about 60°C. Leave for 2–3 min, or until the stain is begining to dry with a blue-green sheen around the edges. Wash the stain off in distilled water, dry and mount in DPX.

H & E–phloxine (for GMA sections)
1. Stain the dried section in Meyer's haematoxylin.   20 min
2. Wash quickly.
3. Differentiate very quickly in 1% acid alcohol.
4. Wash in water.
5. Blue in Scott's tap water or lithium carbonate.   1–2 min
6. Wash.
7. Stain in eosin–phloxine.   5 min

8. Take through three changes of absolute ethanol.   1 min each
9. Clear in two changes of xylene and mount in DPX.

Giemsa resin staining protocol

1. 20% Giemsa stain.   1.5 h 30°C
2. 0.5% acetic acid rinse.
3. 95% ethanol rinse.   Two changes
4. Isopropanol rinse.   Three changes
5. Clear in xylene, and mount in DPX.

Results

Nuclei   Violet
Cytoplasm   Blue
Erythrocytes   Pink

6.5.4 Block staining

Because most stains act by diffusion, they are best suited to thin sections, and only a limited number, chiefly the natural nuclear dyes, are used to stain entire specimens. Both Baker's Haematal 8 and the carmine mixtures given are capable of staining blocks of tissue, from which many stained, thin sections can be rapidly cut and mounted. Impregnation by reduced metal ions, using silver nitrate and gold chloride, have also been used, and the reader is referred to Davenport (1960) for specific methods. A protocol for block staining botanical specimens has been published by Tolbert (1962).

6.5.5 Multiple staining of sections

It is often desirable to compare the distribution of tissues that have been demonstrated using different stains or antibodies. One way to do this, particularly when applying antigens, is to mount multiple sections in the same orientation on a single slide, and treat each differently. Using plastic-coated multi-spot slides, which have a clear spot on which the sections are mounted, is one way to prevent cross-reaction of antisera and stain contamination. The coating does, sometimes, take up stains, so another technique is to use a PAP™ pen to draw a hydrophobic ring around each section before application of the antibody. While the commercially produced multi-spot slides are effective, they are relatively expensive. Eid (1993) has published a simple method, using hydrophobic adhesive tape, to manufacture multi-spot slides; the tape can be removed prior to counterstaining and mounting. A grid of dry DPX mountant, painted onto a clean, grease-free slide will serve the same purpose and, additionally, permit easy alignment of serial sections.

When stains are used on paraffin-embedded sections, it is possible to protect zones with single sections and to stain each sequentially. This obviously works best with two or three reasonably large sections on each slide. Each section is divided off by coating with a layer of wax or grease from one end, leaving the exposed section clear, which is then stained. The remaining zones are then dewaxed and stained before mounting. It is possible to extend this technique to include multiple stains on one section, but it should be remembered that many pathological processes are focal in nature, and may be missed if the section is divided into too many portions.

6.6 Cytological stains

6.6.1 Neutral stains

As well as purely acid or basic dyes, it is possible to create a staining solution from the coloured salt of a mixture of these dyes. These solutions are termed 'neutral' to distinguish them from amphoteric dyes, but this term does not refer to any particular pH. The threefold action of neutral staining solutions results in a powerful single-bath stain for cell components. The R-G stain is an example of a neutral stain which is important for the purple colour that it imparts to nuclei, as distinct from the blue and red colouration of its component dyes—basic Thionin/Azure A and acidic Eosin Y (Wittekind, 1983). These metachromatic stains are used in haematology for pleural and cerebrospinal fluids, and to distinguish parasites in blood films. Because they are mixtures of acidic and basic dyes, the R-G stains are prone to precipitation during use. Some workers (Liao *et al.*, 1982) have suggested additives to improve the stability and shelf-life of these dye mixtures. The stains are diluted from an alcoholic stock with aqueous buffer to liberate the chromophores, and the results depend upon accurate control of pH.

The principal Romanowsky stains are Giemsa, Leishman and Wright. Other similar stains, Jenner and May-Grünwald, contain unripened methylene blue, and are not truly Romanowsky stains but may be combined usefully with those that do contain oxidized methylene blue. Modifications are, nevertheless, slight. The May-Grünwald Giemsa stain is useful for differentiating blood cells and their precursors (Lopes Cardozo, 1977), while Field's stain (Drury and Wallington, 1980) is suitable for examining thick blood films for malarial parasites. Thick, rather than the usual thin, films are advantageous because the parasites (which are often scarce) are thereby concentrated.

Designed for cytological preparations, these stains are susceptible to some variability when applied to tissues, and Giemsa is best suited to staining sections. This phenomenon has been reviewed by Wittekind *et al.* (1991). Secondary fixation for 15–20 min is a prerequisite for good staining; a crisper effect is seen on wet-fixed than air-dried cells. If too much formalin fixation is used, the cells will only stain blue. The stain needs time to develop, and if applied to thick smears will give variable results and also lack purple staining.

It is difficult to standardize the R-G stain because the thiazine component is composed of the oxidation products of methylene blue, in particular Azure B. The precise manner in which a batch will stain depends on the ratios and concentrations of these dyes and, like haematoxylin, the oxidation process is continuous. Nevertheless, it has been shown that the staining action of R-G stains is due to Azure B and eosin. A standardized R-G stain for wet-fixed material, rather than the conventional air-dried and methanol-fixed specimens, has been published by Schulte and Wittekind (1989 a, b).

Standard R-G stain (Wittekind and Kretschmer 1987)
Stock

Azure B-thiocyanate	75 mg
Eosin Y *acid* disodium salt	120 mg
DMSO	100 ml

Dissolve the Azure B in the 75 ml DMSO at 37°C, and the eosin in the remaining 25 ml (DMSO crystalizes below 18°C). Slowly mix the two solutions. This solution will keep in the dark at room temperature for many months, but should not be used if it contains precipitate. To prolong the storage time, and retard oxidation and precipitation, lower to pH 4 by adding hydrochloric acid.

Working solution (1:50)

Stock solution	1 ml
0.03 M Hepes or phosphate buffer pH 6.5	49 ml

Protocol
1. Post-fix air-dried smears or cytospins in methanol or (recommended) the stock solution.   3 min
2. Rinse briefly in distilled water.
3. Stain in the working solution.   15–30 min
4. Rinse in distilled water.
5. Dry in air and mount in DPX.

Differentiation, or de-staining, of R-G-stained cells should be with the diluent methanol, which should be acid-free so that nuclei will subsequently stain purple rather than blue. If the blue colour predominates, the smear may be differentiated by dipping in 0.01% acetic acid. If the smear remains pink, this usually indicates that the pH is wrong. The pH 6.5, rather than pH 7, impedes over-staining—the erythrocytes should be differentiated orange-red. A failure to impart purple in the cell nuclei may be due to the eosin concentration being too low, too much acidic differentiation or insufficient staining. It is important that the smears be thin, otherwise the stain may stain blue overall, without any purple staining. DMSO is a better diluent than the methanol–glycerol mixtures usually quoted. Bone marrow films should be stained with a 1:25 working solution. The Giemsa stain given below can also be applied after the Jenner, Leishman, Wright or May-Grünwald stains alone.

Results
Basiphil cytoplasm:
Polymorphonuclear leucocytes	
Lymphocytes, monocytes	Blue
Plasma cells	
Parasitic protzoa	

Chromatin:
Polymorphonuclear leucocytes	Purple
Lymphocytes, monocytes	
Nucleoli	Light blue
Nuclei of plasma cells	Red
Nuclei of parasitic protzoa	

Acidophil cytoplasm:
Polymorphonuclear leucocytes	Pink
Acidophil granules	
Erythrocytes	Orange-red
Neutrophil granules of cytoplasm of polymorphonuclear leucocytes	
Platelet granules	Purple
Auer rods	
Howell-Jolly bodies	
Connective tissue	
Elastic membranes	Green-blue
Doehle bodies	Bright blue
Toxic bodies	Black

Giemsa stain
Stock
Methylene blue eosinate	4 g
Azure B eosinate	5 g
Azure A eosinate	1 g
Methylene blue chloride	2 g
Glycerol	132 ml
Methanol	132 ml

Two grams of the Giemsa powder are mixed with the glycerol, and heated for 2 h at 60°C. The methanol is then stirred in. When cool, the mixture is shaken and kept in an airtight bottle. It will keep for 3–4 years.

1. Bring the sections to water.
2. Immerse in buffer pH 6.8.   5–10 min

3. Immerse the slides in cold Giemsa working
    solution (diluted 1:10 with buffer)   60 min
    or bring to 60°C (in the wax oven).   30 min
4. Differentiate in buffer until pink, and blot dry.
5. Dehydrate rapidly in *n*-butanol, clear in xylene
    and mount in DPX.

Results

Nuclei	Blue/purple
Mast cell granules	
Basiphil granules	Deep purple
Collagen	
Erythrocytes	
Keratin	Pink
Neutrophil granules	
Eosinophil granules	Scarlet

The best fixative for sections is Helly's fluid. Otherwise formalin or Carnoy's fixative may be used, and if so, the buffer may require reduction to pH 4–5.

6.6.2 Papanicolaou stain

There are several variants of this well-known staining method, which was developed for gynaecological cytology, and depends on a mixture of dyes to differentiate the constituents of cytoplasm, which is amphoteric. The variants are comprehensively described in Boon and Drijver (1985) and a mechanistic review of Papanicolaou's stain has been written by Marshall (1983). Bismark brown Y is often omitted from commercial batches of counterstain, since it is a cationic dye, unlike most other cytoplasmic dyes, and is thought to play no significant part in staining. A few workers include Bismark brown Y believing that it modulates the action of phosphotungstic acid which, in turn, is thought to influence the cytoplasmic staining by the anionic dyes. A modified version of the Papanicolaou stain has been developed (Wittekind *et al.*, 1982), omitting both Orange G and Bismark brown Y and replacing haematoxylin with thionin. It is suggested that this version (not given here) is more reproducible and amenable for automatic screening.

Orange G (OG 6)

Orange G stock 0.5% in 95% ethyl alcohol	100 ml
Phosphotungstic acid	0.015 g

Eosin-azure (EA 50)

Light green SF (yellowish) 0.1% in 45% ethyl alcohol	45 ml
Bismark brown Y 0.5% in 95% ethyl alcohol	10 ml
Eosin (yellowish) 0.5% in 95% ethyl alcohol	45 ml
Phosphotungstic acid	0.2 g
Lithium carbonate (saturated aqueous)	1 drop

The numbers assigned to eosin-azure (30, 50, 65) in the literature (Boon and Drijver, 1985; Coleman and Chapman, 1989) are a code for the proportions of Eosin Y. Fixation is important, and wet-fixed rather than air-dried samples are essential for good results.

Protocol
1. Fix as appropriate and take smears through 80,70 and 50% alcohol to water. If a PEG-based spray fixative has been used, leave the slides in 50% alcohol for at least 1 h or longer.
2. Stain in Harris' or Cole's haematoxylin. 3 min
3. Rinse in tap water. 1–2 min
4. Differentiate in 0.5% aqueous ethanol. Few seconds
5. Rinse in tap water and blue nuclei in Scott's tap water.
6. Rinse in tap water. Few seconds
7. Transfer to 70% then 95% alcohol. Few seconds
8. Stain in OG 6. 3 min
9. Rinse in two changes of 95% alcohol. Few seconds
10. Stain in EA 50 until desired intensity is reached. 2–4 min
11. Rinse in two changes of 95% alcohol. Few seconds
12. Dehydrate, clear and mount in neutral medium.

Results

Nuclei	Dark blue
Cytoplasm of superficial (cornified) cells	Pink
Cytoplasm of intermediate (non-cornified) cells	Pale green-blue
Cytoplasm of parabasal cells	Deep green-blue
Cytoplasm of leucocytes	Pale blue
Cytoplasm of endocervical cell	Blue or green-blue
Erythrocytes	Bright red
Bacteria	Pale blue-grey
Candida (*monila*)	Red
Trichomonads	Grey-green

Some authorities use Harris' haematoxylin at half-strength with omission of the acetic acid, and use it within a few months of manufacture. Mayer's haematoxylin tends to over-oxidize quickly, and preparations thus stained fade more rapidly than when other nuclear stains are used. An acid, rather than acid–alcohol differentiating solution, is less prone to detach cells and cause 'floaters'. Wash the slides thoroughly before restaining, to avoid precipitation of alkaline salts. Two modifications of the differentiation step have been suggested (Soost *et al.*, 1979), to distinguish various states of malignant cell. As with most polychrome staining methods, careful control of the differentiation step is essential for optimum demonstration of the cytoplasm, which should be transparent, yet stained. The eosin-azure counterstain should be well-mixed before use, to give a consistent green result; if allowed to stand the dyes tend to precipitate out of solution. The

Papanicolaou stain was developed empirically, and there are many variations in laboratories worldwide. Automatic staining schedules can be found in Drury and Wallington (1980) and Boon and Drijver (1985), but these must be run, and monitored, with care.

6.7 Polychrome stains

The methods given in the preceding section are both polychrome stains. Papanicolaou's stain is derived from Mallory's trichrome technique (Mallory, 1936) which, together with Johansen's quadruple stain (Johansen, 1939) and Heidenhain's 'Azan' is given here. For other trichrome stains, the reader is referred to Cook (1974) and Culling et al. (1985). Another method (Shoobridge, 1983), a development of Mallory's, is suitable for use with automated staining equipment; the cytoplasmic counterstains are not as vivid as Masson's trichrome, which tends to obscure detail. Everett and Miller (1973) have published a further modification of Mallory's applicable to fetal material.

Other polychrome stains which are applicable to epoxy resins may be found in Jha (1976) and Warmke and Lee (1976), for zoological and botanical tissues, respectively. A further paper by Scala et al. (1993) reports a polychrome technique suitable for acrylic resins. Most of these polychrome stains are empirical, but Davenport (1979) has published a partially histochemical method.

Mallory's triple stain
Solution A
1% (aq) acid fuchsin

Solution B

Aniline blue	0.5 g
Orange G	2.0 g
Phosphomolybdic acid	1.0 g
Distilled water	100 ml

Make up the 1% phosphomolybdic acid solution, dissolve the dyes and filter.

1. Bring the sections to water.
2. Stain with alum haematoxylin-celestine blue.
3. Differentiate in 1% acid alcohol.
4. Wash in running tap water.
5. Stain in 1% (aq) acid fuchsin.   5 min

6. Wash quickly in water.   2 min
7. Stain in solution B.   A few dips
8. Wash in running water, until the water is clear.   15 min

9. Take the slide to 95% ethanol, and differentiate until the section clears from muddy purple to blue and red coloured tissues.
10. Transfer via absolute ethanol to xylene, then xylene saturated with salicylic acid, and mount.

Results

Cartilage	
Fibrous connective tissue	
Amyloid	Blue
Bone ground substance	
Mucin	
Collagen	Deep blue
Muscle	
Fibrin	Red
Axis cylinders	
Nerves	Purple
Glands	
Erythrocytes	
Keratin	Yellow-orange
Myelin	

Tissue may be fixed in 10% neutral-buffered formalin, but brighter results are obtained following primary, or otherwise secondary, fixation in picric acid, dichromate or mercuric chloride-containing fixatives. The hae-matoxylin nuclear stain is optional; if omitted, the nuclei stain red. The blue colour is very rapidly differentiated from the section, and must be controlled microscopically. Loss of the stain may be reduced by dehydrating with *t*-butyl alcohol (2-methylpropan-2-ol). The xylene will arrest leaching of the dye; acidic xylene and an acidic mountant are recommended to reduce fading.

Johansen's quadruple stain

Solution A

Safranin	2.0 g
Methyl cellosolve (ethylene glycol monomethyl ether)	100 ml
50% (aq) ethanol	100 ml
Formaldehyde (mordant)	7.5 ml
Sodium acetate (accentuator)	3.0 g

Solution B

1% (aq) methyl violet 2B (or crystal violet)

Differentiating solution 1

95% (aq) ethanol	30 ml
Methyl cellosolve	30 ml
t-Butyl alcohol	30 ml

Solution C

Methyl cellosolve	6 ml
Clove oil	6 ml

(mix the above, saturate with Fast green FCF (16%) and filter)

95% (aq) ethanol	35 ml
t-Butyl alcohol	35 ml
1% acetic acid	1 ml

Differentiating solution 2

Methyl cellosolve	50 ml
95% (aq) ethanol	50 ml
t-Butyl alcohol	50 ml
Acetic acid (glacial)	0.5 ml

Solution D

Saturated Orange G (12%) in methyl cellosolve	10 ml
Saturated Orange G (12%) in 95% (aq) ethanol	10 ml

(prepare separately and mix)

Methyl cellosolve	20 ml
95% (aq) ethanol	20 ml

Differentiating solution 3

Clove oil	30 ml
Methyl cellosolve	30 ml
95% (aq) ethanol	30 ml

Dehydrating solution

Clove oil	30 ml
Absolute ethanol	30 ml
Xylene	30 ml

1. Bring the sections to 70% ethanol.
2. Stain in Solution A. — 1–3 days
3. Wash in running water, until the water is clear.
4. Stain in Solution B. — 10–15 min
5. Rinse sections in water.
6. Differentiate in Solution 1. — 10–15 sec
7. Stain in Solution C. — 20 min
8. Differentiate in Solution 2. — 5–10 sec
9. Stain in Solution D, until cytoplasm is orange. — 3–5 min
10. Differentiate in Solution 3. — A few dips
11. Rinse in dehydrating solution. — 10–15 sec
12. Rinse in xylene with a trace of absolute ethanol.
13. Take through two changes of xylene and mount.

Results

Chromosomes	Red
Nuclei	Purple

Lignified cell walls	Red
Cellulose walls	Orange-green
Middle lamellae	Green
Collenchyma cells	Yellow-green
Cytoplasm	Orange
Casparian strips	Bright red
Endodermal cell wall	Yellow
Parasitic fungi	Green

The differentiating solutions will need frequent replacement, to ensure crisp staining, which is only apparent after the last differentiation. Prepare Solution C several days in advance: it dissolves slowly. The nuclear staining may be enhanced by additionally using alum haematoxylin before the quadruple stain, but differentiation of the haematoxylin should be minimal. On account of the methyl cellosolve, this technique is not suitable for LVN sections.

Heidenhain's 'Azan'
Solution A
Azocarmine GX or B	0.1 g
Distilled water	100 ml
Acetic acid (glacial)	1 ml

Boil to dissolve the azocarmine, cool, filter, and add the glacial acetic acid.

Solution B
Aniline blue WS	0.5 g
Orange G	2.0 g
8% (aq) acetic acid	100 ml

Dissolve at 50–60°C, cool and filter. Dilute this stock 1:3 with distilled water just prior to use.

1. Take sections to water.
2. Stain with Solution A at 50–60°C in a Coplin jar. 45–60 min
3. Cool, in the stain to room temperature. 15 min
4. Wash in running water. 1 min
5. Differentiate in 0.1% aniline in 95% ethanol. 10–15 sec
6. Rinse in 2% acetic acid to stop differentiation.
7. Wash in running water.
8. Differentiate in 5% phosphotungstic acid in 25% methanol. 30–60 min
9. Wash in running water.
10. Stain in Solution B. 15 min
11. Wash, dehydrate and differentiate in 95% ethanol.
12. Take through two changes of xylene and mount.

Results

Nuclei	
Erythrocytes	Red
Fibrin	
Muscle	Orange-red
Collagen	Blue

The initial differentiation should leave the muscle red, and the collagen pale red.

6.8 Vital stains

If it is possible to stain living cells, why does the microscopist go to the trouble to fix, embed, cut and stain non-living material with all the associated artifacts, especially as phase-contrast techniques permit the study of unstained living material? The answer lies in the fact that vital stains are selective, and unfixed, unstained tissues exhibit poor contrast. Nevertheless, the use of selective stains can be extremely useful as functional probes (Foskett and Grinstein, 1990), and this is the main way in which vital stains are employed, rather than merely to avoid preparation artifacts.

Where stains are applied to living tissues in the body, the process is called *intravital*; where living cells are stained as a slide preparation, the process is termed *supravital*. Vital stains are also used to make cell viability counts, and two such methods involving the use of Nigrosin WS and acridine orange are given below.

Most vital stains are applied at very low concentrations (0.01% w/v) in order to minimize disruption to the material. Supravital preparations must be viewed within an hour of preparation, and the material is then usually thrown away rather than made into a permanent mount, because the cell alters in response to the staining insult. Temporary preparations can be mounted in a physiological solution which must be made up freshly to avoid flocculation. For the same reason, vital stains are kept as 1% or 0.1% stocks, and diluted for use. Other suitable techniques, besides an immersion-stained preparation, are staining by irrigation, or the introduction of the stain using a tissue culture chamber.

Acridine orange
Stocks
0.1% acridine orange in 0.5 M phosphate buffer pH 6.0
1.0% aqueous calcium chloride as differentiator

1. Bring the sections or smears to water.
2. Treat with 1% aqueous acetic acid.   6 sec

3. Wash briefly in distilled water.
4. Stain in acridine orange.   3 min
5. Wash in phosphate buffer.   1 min
6. Differentiate in 10% calcium chloride in distilled water.
7. Mount in phosphate buffer.

Results
Intracellular DNA   }
Collagen, mast cells   }   Green
Intracellular RNA   Red/orange

For a rapid method, combine the acetic acid and acridine orange as an aqueous stain, immerse the smear or section for 10 sec, differentiate in 2% ethanol in physiological saline, rinse and mount in saline. Examine with a fluorescence microscope, using blue light of 460–490 nm. The best results are obtained with fresh, unfixed tissue, although mounted sections may be briefly fixed (about 5 min) in 5% acetic acid in absolute ethanol. Specimens which are fixed after staining in Millonig's glutaraldehyde fixative (Cambier *et al.*, 1977) may be stored for at least 6 months, and exhibit reduced fading and background fluorescence.

Nigrosin WS and neutral red
Both these stains are used as 0.01% solutions in water or buffer. Viable cells exclude Nigrosin WS, while dead or dying cells take up the stain to differing extents. Neutral red is useful for distinguishing macrophages (which take up the stain) from fibroblasts (which do not).

Janus green B
This stain is well-known as a vital stain for mitochondria. It is prepared as a 0.001% solution in ethanol, and a drop allowed to dry on a microscope slide. The cell culture is then applied to the dried stain and a coverslip added. Satisfactory staining will occur in 3–10 min.

6.9 Staining for bacteria

Only the classical methods of Gram and Ziehl-Neelsen will be presented here. For other protocols for bacteria and viral inclusions, the reader is referred to Drury and Wallington (1980) and Clark (1981). The Gram stain divides bacteria into Gram-positive and Gram-negative classes. The former group retain the aniline dye after treatment with iodine, while the latter group are decolourized. The Gram-negative bacteria are visualized with a counterstain. The method depends upon the differential solubility of the trapped alcoholic stain, in different classes of bacteria during differentiation. The iodine acts as a mordant.

It is possible to over-differentiate the stain, particularly in tissue sections which, although thin (3–5 µm), are much thicker than the bacteria, and some organisms may be over-differentiated once the differentiating fluid has penetrated the entire section. Over-differentiation stains Gram-positive bacteria red, and under-differentiation gives a blue result. For this reason, some workers prefer the Gram–Twort modification (Drury and Wallington, 1980).

Gram stain

Crystal violet	2 g
95% ethyl alcohol	20 ml
Ammonium oxalate	0.8 g
Distilled water	80 ml

Dissolve the dye in the alcohol, the ammonium oxalate in the water and mix the two; this solution will be stable for 2 years.

Lugol's iodine mordant

Iodine	1 g
Potassium iodide	2 g
Distilled water	300 ml

Dehydrating solution

Aniline	200 ml
Xylene	100 ml

1. Take sections to water.
2. Stain with crystal violet.   2–3 min
3. Wash off stain with Gram's iodine and leave.   2–3 min
4. Differentiate in absolute alcohol or acetone.
5. Do not rinse, stain directly in 1% (aq) neutral red.   Few seconds
6. Rinse rapidly in water.
7. Blot dry, rapidly dehydrate in solution 3.
8. Clear in xylene and mount.

Results

Gram-positive bacteria	Blue-black
Gram-negative bacteria	Red
Background tissues, some non-viable Gram-positive organisms	Light pink
Background keratin, fibrin, calcium	Blue-grey

Most background tissues are red, but some (e.g. keratin, fibrin and calcium) may be blue-black. The crystal violet (methyl violet 10B) can be replaced with 0.5% (aq) methyl violet 6B, which is differentiated in acetone. The violet dyes methyl, crystal and gentian violet are related via a para-rosanilin structure with various methyl chromatophores, the number of which determine the shade of violet. Two papers on the standardization of the Gram stain are to be found by Bartholomew (1962) and Tucker and Bartholomew (1962). A further paper (Engbæk et al., 1979) reviews other methods for staining bacteria in sections, and suggests a modified method of Brown and Hopps.

Ziehl-Neelsen stain for acid-fast bacteria

Acid-fast bacteria may be stained with the Ziehl-Neelsen technique,which requires heating the section with steaming carbol-fuchsin solution.

Basic fuchsin	1 g
Absolute alcohol	10 ml
5% (aq) phenol	100 ml

Dissolve reagents in the order given.

1. Bring the section to water; stain the section *either* in hot carbol-fuchsin in a Coplin jar for 30 min at 56°C, *or* by covering the section with a small square of filter paper, heating the slide flooded with stain until it steams, and leaving it for 10 min.
2. Wash the section and differentiate in acid alcohol until it is a very pale pink when washed.
3. Wash in water; counterstain in 0.1% methylene blue.
4. Wash, dehydrate and mount in resin.

6.10 Removal of intrinsic pigments

The removal of pigments from sections prior to staining is a specialist subject, and readers will find a chapter devoted to the topic in Drury and Wallington (1980). This section deals with the removal of the more commonly found pigments only. These pigments appear after fixation, and if not washed out of the tissue before embedding, will interfere with subsequent staining.

6.10.1 Formalin and malarial pigments

The fine brown crystals of formalin pigment, which are present in blood-rich tissues that have been stored for a long period in formalin, may be removed as follows. Sections are taken directly from alcohol, and placed in a saturated (8%) solution of picric acid in absolute ethanol for 5–10 min. The section is then washed in running water for 10 min, and the subsequent staining protocols are followed as normal. Formalin pigment is very similar to malarial pigment, seen in erythrocytes of parasitic tissues. Malarial pigment is removed in exactly the same way, and can be distinguished from formalin pigment in that the former is birefringent, while formalin pigment is not.

6.10.2 Mercury pigment

The pigment which results after fixation in fixatives such as Zenker's, SUSA and Helly's can be removed by dissolution in alcoholic iodine. Dewaxed sections are washed in absolute ethanol, and immersed in 0.5% iodine in 70% ethanol for 5 min (with agitation for 2 min). This iodine solution can be re-used, and keeps indefinitely. Following a brief rinse in tap water, the sections are immersed in fresh 5% sodium thiosulphate for up to 2 min, until the sections are bleached. Proceed with staining after a 5 min wash in tap water to remove excess salts from the sections. Baker (1958) showed that Lugol's iodine is less effective for this purpose, since it contains potassium iodide, which dissolves some mercuric chloride protein complexes.

6.10.3 Picric acid

The yellow colour left in tissues stained with fixatives such as Bouin's rarely interferes with staining, but may be removed by immersing the hydrated sections for 30 sec in dilute alkali. Take care not to use too strong an alkali solution in case the sections float off the slide. Traditionally, 0.1% lithium carbonate, which keeps indefinitely and can be re-used once or twice, is used.

6.10.4 Osmium tetroxide

The black deposits of osmium dioxide that form when tissues reduce the tetroxide can be removed by immersing sections for 2–30 min, as required, in 2% fresh aqueous hydrogen peroxide diluted from 30% (100 volumes available oxygen) stock. A 30 min wash in running tap water is needed to remove all traces of fixative.

6.11 Dye purity

The section on haematoxylin gives a rational formula, Haematal 8, developed by Baker, which gives consistent results without the need for differentiation. Unfortunately, such standardized control is not usually possible when staining. Variations in staining occur because manufacturers sell different mixtures (which have different concentrations of active dye and associated impurities) under the same name, all of which may have different shelf lives. Impurities may be other coloured moieties, colourless chemicals or intermediates of dye synthesis. Both inert and reactive impurities can alter the staining characteristics of the dye from one batch, or manufacturer's product, to another.

Rational staining is impeded, too, by confusion over nomenclature, and the mode of action of many dye stuffs. These considerations are listed not to discourage the beginner from even starting to use dyes, but rather to emphasize why for instance there may be over 50 different H & E protocols. Poorly rinsed and washed glassware with contaminating detergents can also influence staining results, causing precipitation of dyes and/or alteration in the pattern or intensity of staining.

Whilst standardization has not procluded the successful use of stains, the rational use of standardized dyes permits better and more consistent staining, and the wider use of automatic staining equipment. It is not feasible to produce very pure dyes economically, because the majority of the market caters not for the biologist, but for the textile industry. The single most important barrier to the production of analytical grade dyes, however, is the isolation and characterization of the individual components in what is a very complex mixture. Purifying large quantities of ionized dyes is difficult when the ionic components adsorb easily onto the carrier substratum.

The Biological Stain Commission assays commercial dyes, and certifies those which perform well in routine tests and which meet certain physicochemical standards (Lillie, 1977), and the European Committee for Clinical Laboratory Standards has reported in the *Histochemical Journal* (1992) on dye standards for several specific dyes. There is also an excellent review of standardization in biological staining by Schulte (1991).

The best practical advice is first to use only those stains which have been certified, and to note the batch number of the relevant dye. About 60 dyes are now routinely certified, and all reputable manufacturers submit their products for certification before sale, although staining solutions of dyes are not certified. Secondly, where it is crucial to eliminate a false result (positive or negative) from a particular staining technique, it is usual to take a known positive control through the protocol. Suitable control tissues are listed in Appendix 4 of Bancroft and Cook (1984).

References

Baker JR. (1958) *Principles of Biological Microtechnique: a Study of Fixation and Dyeing.* Methuen, London.

Baker JR. (1964) A substitute for Ehrlich's haematoxylin and similar dyes used in biological microtechnique. *School Sci. Rev.* **45**, 400–401.

Baker JR, Jordan BM. (1953) Miscellaneous contributions to microtechnique. *Q. J. Microscop. Sci.* **94**, 237–242.

Bancroft JD, Cook HC. (1984) *Manual of Histological Techniques.* Churchill Livingstone, Edinburgh.

Bartholomew J. (1962) Variables influencing results, and the precise definition of steps in Gram staining as a means of standardizing the results obtained. *Stain Technol.* **37**, 139–155.

Boon ME, Drijver JS. (1985) *Routine Cytological Staining Techniques: Theoretical Background and Practice*. Macmillan Press Ltd, Basingstoke.

Bradbury S. (1973) *Peacock's Elementary Microtechnique*, 4th revised edn. Edward Arnold, London.

Cambier MA, Wheeless LL, Patten SF. (1977) A new post-staining fixation technique for acridine orange. *Acta Cytol.* **21**, 477.

del Cerro M, Standler NS, del Cerro C. (1980) High resolution optical microscopy of animal tissues by the use of sub-micrometer thick sections and a new stain. *Microscop. Acta* **83**, 217–220.

Clark G. (1979) Displacement. *Stain Technol.* **54**, 111–119.

Clark G. (1981) *Staining Procedures*, 4th edn. Biological Staining Commission, William & Wilkins, Baltimore.

Clark G, Kasten FH. (1973) *History of Staining*, 3rd edn. Williams & Wilkins, Baltimore.

Coleman DV, Chapman PA. (eds) (1989) *Clinical Cytotechnology*. Butterworths, London.

Cook HC. (1974) *Manual of Histological Demonstration Techniques*. Butterworths, London.

Culling CFA, Allison RT, Barr WT. (1985) *Cellular Pathology Technique*, 4th edn. Butterworths, London.

Davenport HA. (1960) *Histological and Histochemical Technics*. WB Saunders, Philadelphia, PA.

Davenport WD Jr (1979) A rapid trichrome staining procedure for the identification of tissue types. *Histochem. J.* **11**, 367–369.

Drury RAB, Wallington EA. (1980) *Carleton's Histological Technique*, 5th edn. Oxford University Press, Oxford.

Eid T. (1993) The use of hydrophobic tape to produce minature wells on microscope slides. *Biotechnic and Histochem.* **68**, 189–192.

Engbæk K, Johansen KS, Jensen ME. (1979) A new technique for Gram staining paraffin-embedded tissue. *J. Clin. Pathol.* **32**, 187–190.

European Committee for Clinical Laboratory Standards. (1992) Dye Standards, Part I & II: terminology and general principles, selected dyes. *Histochem. J.* **24**, 217–242.

Everett MM, Miller WA. (1973) Adaptation of Mallory's trichrome stain to embryonic and fetal material. *Stain Technol.* **48**, 5–7.

Foskett JK, Grinstein S. (1990) *Noninvasive Techniques in Cell Biology*. Wiley–Liss, New York.

Gill GW, Frost JK, Miller KA. (1974) A new formula for a half-oxidized hematoxylin solution that neither overstains nor requires differentiation. *Acta Cytol.* **18**, 300–311.

Gray P. (1954) *The Microtomist's Formulary and Guide*. Blakiston, New York.

Hayat MA. (1975) *Positive Staining for Electron Microscopy*. van Nostrand-Reinhold, New York.

Horobin RW. (1982) *Histochemistry: an Explanatory Outline of Histochemistry and Biophysical Staining*. Gustav Fischer Verlag, Stuttgart; Butterworths, London.

Horobin RW. (1988) *Understanding Histochemistry: Selection, Evaluation and Design of Biological Stains*. Ellis Horwood, Chichester.

Horobin RW. (1990) Understanding stains for light and electron microscopy. *Microsc. Anal.* **18**, 13–15.

Horobin RW, Gerrits PO, Wright DJ. (1990) Staining sections of water-miscible resins. 2. Effects of staining reagent lipophilicity on the staining of glycol-methacrylate-embedded tissues. *J. Microsc.* **166**, 199–205.

Jha RK. (1976) An improved polychrome staining method for thick epoxy sections. *Stain Technol.* **51**, 159–162.

Johansen DA. (1939) A quadruple stain combination for plant tissues. *Stain Technol.* **14**, 125–128.

Kiernan JA. (1990) *Histological & Histochemical Methods: Theory & Practice*, 2nd edn. Pergamon Press, Oxford.

Liao JC, Ponzo JL, Patel C. (1982) Improved stability of methanolic Wright's stain solution with dual additives. *Stain Technol.* **57**, 23–30.

Lillie RD. (1977) *H.J. Conn's Biological Stains*, 9th edn. Williams & Wilkins, Baltimore, MD.

Lillie RD, Pizzolato P, Donaldson PT. (1975) Hematoxylin substitutes: a survey of mordant dyes tested and consideration of the relation of their structure to performance as nuclear stains. *Stain Technol.* **51**, 25–41.

Lopes Cardozo P. (1977) *Atlas of Clinical Cytology*. Lippincott, Philadelphia.

Mallory FB. (1936) The aniline blue collagen stain. *Stain Technol.* **11**, 101–102.

Marshall PN. (1983) Papanicolaou staining—a review. *Microscop. Acta* **87**, 233–243.

Scala C, Preda P, Cenacchi G, Martinelli GN, Manara GC, Pasquinelli G. (1993) A new polychrome stain and simultaneous methods of histological, histochemical and immunohistochemical stainings performed on semithin sections of Bioacryl-embedded human tissues. *Histochem. J.* **25**, 670–677.

Schulte EKW. (1991) Standardization of biological dyes and stains: pitfalls and possibilities. *Histochemistry* **95**, 319–328.

Schulte EKW, Wittekind DH. (1989a) A quick and standardized Giemsa stain for wet-fixed cytological material. *Stain Technol.* **64**, 253–254.

Schulte EKW, Wittekind DH. (1989b) Standardized Thionin-Eosin Y: a quick stain for cytology. *Stain Technol.* **64**, 255–256.

Shoobridge MPK. (1983) A new principle in polychrome staining: a system of automated staining, complementary to haematoxylin and eosin, and useable as a research tool. *Stain Technol.* **58**, 245–258.

Snoek H. (1983) Modification of staining techniques for plant sections. *Microscopy* **34**, 554.

Soost H-J, Falter EW, Otto K. (1979) Comparison of two Papanicolaou staining procedures for automated screening. *Anal. Quant. Cytol.* **1**, 37–42.

Stevens A. (1990) The haematoxylins. In *Theory and Practice of Histological Techniques*, 3rd edn (eds JD Bancroft and A Stevens). Churchill Livingstone, Edinburgh, pp. 109–121.

Tolbert RJ. (1962) Block staining of botanical materials. *Stain Technol.* **37**, 165–169.

Tucker FL, Bartholomew J. (1962) Variations in the Gram staining results caused by air moisture. *Stain Technol.* **37**, 157–160.

Warmke HE, Lee S-LJ. (1976) Improved staining procedures for semithin epoxy sections of plant tissues. *Stain Technol.* **51**, 179–185.

Wittekind DH. (1983) On the nature of Romanowsky-Giemsa staining and its significance for cytochemistry and histochemistry: an overall view. *Histochem. J.* **15**, 1029–1047.

Wittekind D, Kretschmer V. (1987) On the nature of Romanowsky-Giemsa staining and the Romanowsky-Giemsa effect. II. A revised Romanowsky-Giemsa staining procedure. *Histochem J.* **19**, 399–401.

Wittekind D, Hilgarth M, Kretschmer V, Seiffert W, Zipfel E. (1982) A new and reproducible Papanicolaou stain. *Anal. Quant. Cytol.* **4**, 286–294.

Wittekind D, Schulte EKW, Schmidt G, Frank G. (1991) The standard Romanowsky-Giemsa stain in histology. *Biotechnic Histochem.* **66**, 282–295.

7 Finishing the Preparation

7.1 Mountants

Once stained, the preparation must be suitably mounted before it can be studied. The mounting medium serves three purposes.

1. The fluid, gel or solid fills out the spaces between tissue and coverglass so that no air gaps remain to obscure the tissue.
2. It allows the contrast of the preparation to be adjusted, and thus emphasizes the detail of the specimen.
3. It provides a permanent seal for the preparation against entry of air, and guards to some extent against mechanical damage.

Mounting media differ according to whether they are used to mount stained or unstained tissues. In the former case, it is important that the medium has a RI as close to that of glass as possible so that the detail demonstrated by the stain can be seen clearly without interference. Where the specimen or tissue is unstained, the RI of the mounting medium should differ from that of the tissue as much as possible. In this way the medium is used to enhance tissue detail that would otherwise be lost. Aqueous mountants are generally of lower RI than resinous formulations.

7.2 Water-based media

Apathy's medium (RI = 1.52)

Gum arabic	30 g
Laevulose	30 g
Distilled water	30 ml

This is a gum sugar formulation. Farrants' medium, the other well-known mixture, is made with glycerol. Gray (1954) states that 'much grief' may be avoided by reducing the water to 20 ml, and using laevulose syrup instead of the dry sugar.

Farrants' medium (RI = 1.42)

Gum arabic	40 g
Glycerol	20 ml
Distilled water	40 ml
Phenol crystals or	0.5 g
10% formalin (preservatives)	1 ml

Glycerol jelly (RI = 1.44–1.47)

Gelatin	10 g
Glycerol	70 ml
Distilled water	60 ml
Thymol (preservative)	One small crystal

Use top-quality bacteriological gelatin to give a water-white solution. Gelatin of 300 bloom is suitable; the higher the bloom number, the tougher the solid gel. Dissolve the gelatin with gentle heat under 40°C, and add the other reagents. Do not use phenol as a preservative, since it may cause stains to fade. Use a water-bath to melt the jelly: direct dry heat will cause minute air bubbles to form in the mixture. If the jelly is cloudy, soak it overnight, drain off the water, melt at 40°C and add two egg whites. Mix thoroughly, and raise the temperature until the egg whites are coagulated. Cool, but do not stir, and strain the mixture through two layers of fine muslin. If the gelatin is overheated, it will break down to metagelatin and will not set; this also occurs if the gelatin is held in liquid form for more than 1 week.

Some media are less suited for particular stains than others because they allow stains to fade or leach out of the preparation. Similarly, stains and dyes should not dissolve into the mountant. For this reason, protocols call for water-based mountants where fat stains, or some histochemical substrates are employed. Most of these requirements are met by resin-based media. As a consequence, preparations are once again dehydrated and passed through transition or clearing fluids before mounting in media which are water-immiscible.

7.3 Dehydration and clearing

For most routine procedures, this is merely a repeat of the procedure explained under the same heading in Chapter 3 on tissue processing. Usually, the slides are agitated for 1 min in each of 70%, 95% and two changes of 100% ethanol. Avoid going too rapidly into absolute alcohol: this may distort the tissue, and will certainly contaminate the absolute alcohols sooner than expected. With delicate or friable tissue, use initial baths of 50% or even 30% alcohol, with an intermediate bath of 80% alcohol.

If, however, the stain is one that is easily extracted by alcohol, either use an aqueous mountant, or drain off the slides before passing through the alcohols for a few seconds each. Some cationic dyes are much less soluble in *n*-butanol (butan-1-ol) than ethanol; the slides can be well drained—or blotted if the tissue will not suffer—and cleared in two changes of *n*-butanol followed by two or three changes of xylene. Some workers, particularly where *n*-butanol is used for celloidin or LVN sections, take the sections through an equal mixture of *n*-butanol and xylene before the xylene. An alternative is to use acetone or isopropyl alcohol (propan-2-ol) as the dehydrant, since acetone will not leach methyl blue or other thiazo dyes from solution. Acetone does, however, dissolve celloidin and LVN from sections, as will isopropanol to some extent. Ethanol does not affect celloidin.

Most routine work calls for transfer from the second absolute alcohol straight into the transition medium. The alcohols and xylene should be kept fresh; if a milkiness is seen on transferring the slides into xylene, contamination with traces of water, (signalling incomplete dehydration) has occurred, and the slides must be taken back into absolute alcohol. Some workers prefer to use an equal mixture of alcohol–xylene, while others substitute toluene for xylene. Toluene and cedarwood oil are often used as alternative transition media before embedding for delicate specimens; toluene has no advantage over xylene here, but merely evaporates from the slide faster, with the consequent risk of drying the specimen before mounting is completed.

Celloidin sections can either be attached to the slide, or taken as loose sections through the staining reagents. The aniline dyes, which stain the celloidin background, can be removed using 2% colophonium (pine rosin) in 95% alcohol.

7.4 Resinous media

Canada balsam (RI = 1.52)
Derived from the gum of the Canadian fir tree *Abies balsamea*, the classic medium used for many years was Canada balsam dissolved in xylene. This is, however, prone to yellowing with age and oxidizing to form annual rings. It is possible to add anti-oxidants and ring the preparation to prevent this (Section 7.9). Canada balsam tends to be acid, and under these conditions basic aniline counterstains and haematoxylin, in any mounting medium, will fade.

DPX (RI = 1.52)
Canada balsam has been largely replaced by the synthetic resin DPX formulated by Kirkpatrick and Lendrum in 1941. Because far more solvent evaporates from this medium than natural resins, plasticizers such as

dibutyl phthalate are added to prevent the formation of air spaces in the mount.

Euparal (RI = 1.48)

This medium is used where tissues have to be mounted directly from alcohol without passing through xylene or other transition medium. Euparal vert is green, and will preserve the colour of haematoxylin better than colourless Euparal.

Light-polymerizing resin media do not require the use of dangerous solvents, and therefore do not pose the same problems of solvent evaporation and tissue shrinkage as do conventional media. Curing of the resin can be controlled, and time allowed to eject air bubbles. Silverman (1986) reports on the use of two methacrylate plastics which do not cause fading and are not fluorescent.

7.5 Mounting technique

Lay out up to 12 coverslips at a time on a slide tray. Check that they are clean and free from cracks or blemishes. Using a wide disposable pipette or glass dropper, spread a single thick trail of mountant slowly down the length of the coverslip. This action must be done slowly to exclude air bubbles from the mountant. Square or circular coverslips are covered with a drop of the appropriate size. All this is learnt by trial and error; the knack is to include enough mountant to reach the edges of the coverslip when it is pressed into position, yet not have too much mountant that the excess oozes onto fingers, the top of the preparation and everywhere else at once. Nor should there be too little, forming an imperfect seal, that admits air under the coverslip as the solvent evaporates from the mountant.

Replace the glass dropping stick slowly into the bottle of mounting medium so that air is not incorporated into the mass for the next time. It is difficult to remove air bubbles from some media such as XAM, which is similar to DPX. Under these circumstances, it may be helpful to reduce the viscosity of the medium by very gentle warming. This method is to be preferred to thinning by adding excess solvent, which merely leaves an insignificant amount of mountant in solution. In this case, when the solvent evaporates, air is drawn into the preparation.

Using slide forceps, remove the slide from the water or transition medium and drain off the excess, onto a lint-free paper towel. Wipe the back of the slide rapidly, then wipe carefully around the section leaving a margin of fluid around its entirety. The slide is then rapidly inverted, the specimen touched to the mountant, and the slide left to adhere under its own weight. Before the mountant oozes out from the edge of the coverslip turn the slide rightway up again, check for any residual air bubbles, and put in a dust-free place to dry. Air bubbles should be teased out as soon as possible before the mountant becomes too viscous to allow them to be pressed to the edge of the coverslip with a wooden orange stick or the edge of a pencil. Do not use the tip of a pair of forceps, which can crack the coverglass and ruin the preparation.

Mounting preparations from xylene, or other transition media must be done in a fume hood, and the slides left in the fume hood to dry before being labelled and hardened permanently in a 40°C oven for a few days prior to storage in a slide cabinet. It is inadvisable to try to clean the excess mountant, or wipe the top of any coverslip that becomes smeared too soon, since such a smear will be difficult to remove until the preparation is dry. Where DPX or a resin medium is used, the dried mounting medium can be stripped carefully from the slide with the aid of a sharp blade. It is more difficult to clean smeared coverslips of aqueous mounts, since most of these never fully set, and the coverslip has to be held by one corner whilst being swabbed with a saturated tissue.

Where large, thick specimens have been mounted, the risk of air entering under the coverslip as the preparation dries is increased. In these cases, thicker resin solutions should be used to lower the viscosity, and DPX should be avoided because it is viscous even at low concentrations. The usual solvent for resin media is xylene because of its wide use as a transition medium, and its relatively high boiling point. A small lead weight or folded paper-clip will often help to exclude air, particularly from thick gelatin or resin sections. How to fold such a clip is shown in *Figure 7.1*.

7.6 Coverslip thickness

The coverslip is used to protect the specimen; it is important, too, what thickness of coverslip is used to make the preparation. Light is refracted

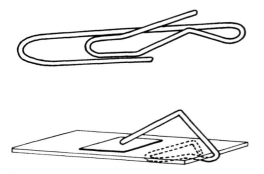

Figure 7.1:   The paper-clip 'weight'. Top: version devised by Mr L. Larkman (with permission from the Postal Microscopical Society). Bottom: an alternative form, which may be seen in use in *Figure 5.9*. It is safer to use than the traditional lead weight (which if preferred for use can be covered in tape).

at the glass–air interface causing rays to be bent; the object appears to originate from different positions with respect to the coverslip, according to the obliquity of the rays. The effect is the same as viewing a stick inserted into water, which appears bent to the observer.

The spherical aberration so caused can be corrected in the objective design for specified coverslip thicknesses. This is internationally set at 0.17 mm, but may be 0.18 mm for some old American and British objectives. The effect is particularly noticeable with dry objectives of high numerical aperture. Theoretically, in a truly homogenous immersion system rays are not refracted from their path, but no immersion system is so exact, and whilst the effect is much reduced, spherical aberration will still occur when coverslips of an incorrect thickness are used. The use of an incorrect immersion medium will worsen this effect also.

The effect of coverslip thickness is negligible for objectives of numerical aperture less than 0.5 NA; objectives over 0.8 NA are so sensitive that it is imperative to correct for aberration when using such an objective for demanding work. Correction may be made by altering the mechanical tubelength by means of a draw-tube (if fitted). The tubelength is shortened (thereby introducing under-corrected spherical aberration) from the standard 160 mm to correct for a thick coverslip, and lengthened to correct for a thin coverslip. A useful summary is given in White (1974). There are some multi-immersion objectives which have a collar similar to the correction collar found on 'high dry' objectives. The function of these collars is the same: the spacing of the internal lens elements of the objective is altered to correct for spherical aberration depending on the coverslip thickness or the immersion medium used.

A binocular instrument does not permit the use of a draw-tube, and so a correction collar must be used, and these are usually only fitted to objectives over 0.9 NA. Setterington (1953) has therefore calculated coverslip tolerances based on an objective of 0.85 NA as a limiting case. The Royal Microscopical Society recommends a tolerance limit of ± 3 µm about the 170 µm standard, with the relaxed specification being ± 6 µm. The coverslip tolerance figures in *Table 7.1* are taken from Pluta (1988), and show the admissible deviation, in millimeters, from the standard for any stated numerical aperture of Zeiss (Oberkochen) objectives. The industry ranges for different standard coverslip thicknesses are also shown.

For really exacting work of the highest standard (for example photomicrography for publication, or for work demanding the use of dry objectives of high numerical aperture), it is best to measure the coverslip to be used with a micrometer gauge. Square or oblong coverslips ought to be measured at both the centre and corners, while circular coverslips, unless really large, need only be measured at the centre.

Previous studies have shown that there is a considerable range of variation amongst the coverslips in any box from the nominal thickness quoted. Spinnell and Loveland (1959) found that as few as 51% of coverslips were within ± 6 µm of the standard thickness, and that the greatest

Table 7.1: Tolerances for coverslip thickness

Coverslip thickness	Industrial range (mm)
No. 0	0.085–0.130
No. 1	0.130–0.160
No. 1½	0.160–0.190
No. 2	0.190–0.250
No. 3	0.250–0.350

Numerical aperture (objective)	Admissible deviation from 0.17 mm (mm)	Total allowed range (mm)
0.08–0.30	0.15	0–0.3
0.31–0.45	0.07	0.10–0.24
0.46–0.55	0.05	0.12–0.22
0.56–0.65	0.03	0.14–0.20
0.66–0.75	0.02	0.15–0.19
0.76–0.85	0.01	0.16–0.18
0.86–0.95	0.005	0.165–0.175

Data taken from Rawlins (1992), p. 57, Table 6.3, with permission from BIOS Scientific Publishers; and Pluta (1988), p. 233, Table 2.9 with permission from Elsevier, Amsterdam and the author.

variation occurred within, rather than between, boxes of 100 pieces. Other studies (Bradbury, 1969; Thornton *et al.*, 1985) have confirmed these findings, and have shown that the thickness range of No. 1½ coverslips is often bi-modal, around 0.18 mm (the old standard) rather than the current international standard of 0.17 mm.

For the use of a measured coverslip to have any meaning the specimen must be mounted directly onto the coverslip, and the specimen weighted during the drying time after mounting. It is possible to buy coverslip staining racks which will take 22 × 22 mm coverslips. Alternatively, use a Columbia jar to stain 22 × 22 mm coverslips.

Two separate studies have been carried out to determine the thickness of mountant usually present between the specimen and coverslip (Aumonier and Setterington, 1967; Woolfe, 1983). In each case 12 slides were studied. The thickness of mountant (which ought to be non-existent with a coverslip of correct thickness) ranged from 10 to 76 μm. On average, the thickess of the mountant above the section was 32 μm, and the combined thickness of coverslip and mountant 19% more than the standard 170 μm. If coverslips are not measured and sections mounted directly upon them, it pays to use No.1 thickness coverslips, with a thin layer of mountant.

Not only must the specimen be mounted in contact with the underside of the coverslip, but it must be less than 6 μm thick, the relaxed RMS standard, as a maximum value for exacting work. The RI must lie within 1.5233–1.5247, and Setterington (1953) notes that this tolerance may be exceeded by a change in temperature of ± 2°C from the standard 20°C.

7.7 Adhesives

Most paraffin sections are routinely dried for 10–30 min onto the microscope slide at a temperature close to the melting point of the wax mixture in use (60°C), but poorly fixed, tough or friable sections will benefit from overnight drying at room temperature or 37°C. The sections should be protected from airborne contaminants whilst drying, preferably in an enclosed oven.

Where there is a danger of sections becoming detached during processing, it is advisable to use an adhesive, as it is much more difficult to mount dislodged sections, or glue down those that have become partly detached. In most cases, adequate drying of the sections on the slide or coverslip is sufficient to prevent detachment. If the protocol calls for treatment with alkali or hot reagents, or the tissues are impregnated with ester wax or a resin, then it is advisable to use an adhesive. This also holds true for most thick serial sections, and the following tissues which have a tendency to detach: neural (especially brain and spinal cord), blood clots, decalcified tissue and those fixed in strong protein coagulants.

Mayer's albumen is the classical adhesive, a very thin smear being applied with the ball of the thumb across the slide. Natural adhesives such as albumen, glycerol and starch may take up dyes, particularly if unevenly applied; 1% methyl cellulose will not do so. Haupt's gelatin is useful for frozen sections (Bissing, 1974). For reviews of modern aqueous, non-aqueous and contact adhesives see Fink (1978a,b,c).

Resin sections can be affixed using a celloidin (cellulose nitrate, LVN) solution, and Fink recommends a 2–10% solution in ethyl, isopropyl, amyl or *tert*-butyl acetate. This mixture can also be used for paraffin and cryostat sections; sections should be soaked in 0.5–1% ether in alcohol after the 100% alcohol rehydration step. For PEG sections use 5% poly-isobutylene in petroleum ether.

The last group worth mentioning are the silane-based adhesives. 3-amino-propyl tri-ethoxy silane (TESPA) is used to coat glass with amino groups that enhance the binding of proteins. As such these coated coverslips are suitable for tissue culture work. One protocol calls for 10% silane in DMSO. Care should be taken while adding the silane to the DMSO diluent. The slides or coverslips are boiled under reflux, using a water-cooled condenser for 1 h at 160°C. The glassware can then be cooled, washed in double-distilled water and dried on Postlip absorbent paper folded into a zig-zag pattern in a dust-free atmosphere.

TESPA-treated / silane-coated coverslips
1. Boil 13 mm coverslips in concentrated nitric acid and
   with anti-bumping granules. Do this in the fume hood.   5 min
2. Wash in two changes of double-distilled water.

3. Transfer to a round-bottomed flask, add 10% silane in DMSO (5 ml silane in 45 ml DMSO).
4. Reflux at 160°C, heating in a glycerol bath (e.g. deep fat fryer).   1 h
5. Wash in three changes of DMSO.
6. Wash several times in double-distilled water, and leave overnight in the penultimate rinse.
7. Rinse again.
8. Dry in a Petri dish lid on a fluted filter paper.
9. Sterilize under UV if required.   1 h

The extractor of the fume hood will lower the efficiency of the Bunsen: switch on the hood once the acid is boiling well, and starts to fume.

A simpler protocol calls for 2% TESPA in acetone. The slides are dipped in their racks, as for the gelatin coating methods, and briefly rinsed in two staining baths of acetone, followed by two further staining baths of distilled water. They are then left to dry in the racks. TESPA-treated slides are only effective for aldehyde-fixed tissues.

Formvar is commonly used as a substrate to support electron microscope ultra-thin sections, but is useful as an adhesive where celloidin might cause background staining, such as in immunology. It is possible to use Formvar to retain acrylic resin sections (LR White) on glass microscope slides. Clean slides are dipped in 2% Formvar in chloroform and dried horizontally. The sections are cut and dried onto the slide at 50°C.

7.7.1 Lifting of sections

GMA sections are prone to lifting when treated with caustic or alcoholic solutions, and when hard tissues are subjected to lengthy staining and washing protocols. Alcian blue 8GX potently renders glass surfaces cationic. Slides are pre-cleaned in 1 M sodium hydroxide for 18 h, followed by 1 M hydrochloric acid for 1 h and absolute ethanol for 15 min at room temperature, with a hot water wash in between each treatment. The slides are then soaked in filtered 0.5% Alcian blue 8GX at 65°C for 15 min, followed by a distilled water wash. The slides are then air-dried for 6–8 h, rinsed in absolute ethanol for 30 sec and air-dried overnight.

Using one of the cleaning methods described below, slides should first be cleaned of any grease before mounting sections. If a thin film of grease is left on the slide when the section is mounted, this will dissolve in the clearing medium and loosen the section. It is not a good idea to use detergents to clean slides, as these not only reduce the surface tension of the cleaning water, so allowing grease to remain undetected, but they may also cause background staining and interference with fluorescence. If it is not possible to use a suitable non-protein adhesive (e.g. silane), sections may be hardened after mounting and before further treatment by drying in 10% formalin vapour in a bell jar.

If, after using appropriately cleaned slides and suitable adhesives, sections still persist in lifting try the following remedies.

(i)   Reduce the use of any alkali in the protocol.
(ii)   Reduce washings if possible, and agitate very gently whilst so doing.
(iii)   Use double-dipped 5% gelatin slides.

Wax sections can be coated in celloidin before staining, as follows, if previous experience indicates a risk of sections lifting.

1.   Dissolve the wax in xylene, and take to absolute ethanol.
2.   Take through an equal mixture of absolute ethanol and ether.
3.   Transfer to 1% celloidin in ethanol and ether in equal proportions.
4.   Remove the slide and part-dry in air; before absolutely dry, transfer to 75% ethanol to gel the celloidin.
5.   Take the slide to water and proceed with staining.

If celloidin is apparent in the stained section, bring the section quickly through an equal mixture of ether–ethanol after the first absolute alcohol, then into the second absolute alcohol and through transition media as usual prior to mounting.

7.8 Cleaning slides

Most good microscopical glassware comes pre-washed, and for most purposes it is sufficient merely to remove any residual surface grease or dust to permit adhesion. A good quality non-gritty scouring powder, mixed into a thin cream with water, will serve most general purposes. Rub the slides with clean fingers, rinse off excess under running water, and finish by drying and polishing with a lint-free cloth.

Alternatively, clean the slides and coverslips in 1% hydrochloric acid in 70% alcohol, and wipe dry with a clean lint-free cloth. Some workers prefer to store their slides in absolute or acid alcohol, and remove them when required. Rinse twice in single distilled water, wash individually in 25% Teepol detergent in distilled water and wash in running distilled water. Dehydrate via an alcohol series to absolute alcohol over 5 min, followed by a similar rehydration to remove any last traces of grease or organic material. Dry the slides briefly on a hot-plate, or in an oven, before use. Another method is to boil the glassware in concentrated nitric acid for 2 min, and wash thoroughly several times in double-distilled water afterwards. Coverslips can conveniently be held within the coils of a suitably gentle spring whilst boiling in acid.

The classical method for cleaning slides is to soak them in potassium dichromate in sulphuric acid. When using any water-based cleaning method which is to be followed by an organic adhesive, clean glassware should be heated over a bunsen to evaporate the surface moisture before dipping.

Dichromate–sulphuric
The classical mixture for cleaning to a high standard requires *great care* in its preparation. To 100 ml saturated aqueous potassium dichromate (about 15–20%) add 150 ml concentrated sulphuric acid. Wash the slides several times in running water finishing with two distilled water washes. Use the solution for as long as potassium dichromate crystals remain in the bottom of the container. Bradbury (1973) gives a simpler formula.

Potassium dichromate (3% aq)   90 ml
Concentrated sulphuric acid   10 ml

Add the sulphuric acid to the potassium dichromate with care, as before.

7.9 Fading of specimens

All coloured preparations undergo fading with time. This results in loss of contrast, and is often irreversible. In some cases, however, it may be possible to remove the coverslip and re-stain. The problem is most acute in sections, where a large surface area to volume ratio is exposed to light. Fading is also a particular problem with fluorochromed sections, and special media have been developed to minimize the fading of such preparations.

Studies have been carried out on the influence of sunlight (Barr, 1970) and artificial light (Lillie *et al.*, 1950, 1953) on the effect of various mounting media. Sections mounted in Canada balsam tended to fade about 30% after 10 h intermittent exposure to sunlight, Dammar xylene by about 20%, Euparal by 25%, DPX by 35% and XAM by 25%. These figures were measured at the maximum optical density for H & E (536 nm). Another study has been conducted (Schmolke, 1993) on sections embedded in epoxy resin and stored in the dark. In this study, Eukitt-mounted (48%) and unmounted sections faded the most (38%), compared to those mounted in DPX (13%). Canada balsam and other natural resins contain acids and unsaturated reducing agents which cause fading. Euparal vert conserves the staining of haematoxylin, due to the presence of copper salts. The colourless Euparal variant was recommended for Romanowsky stains, since mounting can be performed directly from 90% alcohol; others have suggested Diaphane, a similar medium to Euparal, for the same purpose. The RI of both media is 1.483, which is lower than that of Canada balsam.

Paraffin crystallizes in DPX, but not in balsam, if the same xylene is used for dewaxing and dehydrating the sections. Prussian blue, which fades very rapidly in acid mountants, such as Canada balsam, is retained well in DPX. Most synthetic media 'craze' with the production of annual rings from oxidation of the mountant (Hollander and Frost, 1970), and cause fading of stains, particularly the basiphilic (e.g. Romanowsky) types. For this reason, some authorities propose that resin-mounted slides should be ringed with two shellac finishing coats, in a similar manner to fluid mounts. Hollander and Frost (1971), successfully used 1% 2-6-di-*tert*-butyl-*p*-cresol as an anti-oxidant in resinous mounting media. Another anti-oxidant, *p*-phenylenediamine has been used for retarding the fading of fluorescent stains, and is discussed below.

7.9.1 Sections stained with fluorochromes

Where measurement of fluorescence intensity is important, it is essential to retard fading and take photomicrographs as soon as possible. Fading is proportional to the intensity of the excitation. Powerful reducing agents are used to retard fluorescence fading caused by free oxygen radicals or the excited states of dyes. Glycerol retards fluorescence fading, and is used as a component of most formulae. Johnson *et al.* (1981) recommend the use of 0.1% (w/v) *p*-phenylenediamine added to 10 ml phosphate-buffered saline pH 7.4 (0.01 M PO_4 in 0.15 M NaCl) in 90 ml of glycerol. A review of other suitable additives, and the phenomenon of fluorescence fading, is given by Johnson *et al.* (1982) and Valnes and Brandtzaeg (1985).

The use of β-mercaptoethanol as a 0.02% solution (v/v) in DPX has been investigated for several fluorochromes (Franklin & Fillion, 1985). The authors stress that unless slides were thoroughly dried, preferably over a vacuum dessicator overnight, quenching of fluorescence occurred. A further simple recipe based on the active ingredients 1,4-diazo-bicyclo-(2,2,2)-octane (DABCO) and polyvinyl alcohol (gelvatol) is given below.

1. To 40 ml 0.02 M PO_4 buffer at pH 7.2, add 0.14 M NaCl.
2. Add sodium azide as a preservative at 0.04% final concentration.
3. Cover the beaker with foil to prevent the entry of light; weigh out 1% DABCO (sticky) directly into the beaker.
4. Add 10 g gelvatol, and stir overnight, with a magnetic stirrer, for about 16 h.
5. Check dissolution, add 20 ml glycerol and stir overnight again.
6. Check pH to about 6–7.
7. Spin at 30 000 g for 15 min.
8. Divide into aliquots in light-tight tubes, store at 4°C.

7.10 Finishing the preparation

Fluid and gelatin mounts need to be sealed against evaporation, entry of air and mechanical damage, as they do not set hard in the same way as plastic- or resin-mounted preparations. Even these latter preparations benefit from a sealing ring of lacquer to prevent leakage and oxidation, and to protect the mount. A ringing table is useful not only for applying finishing coats of varnish to a preparation, but also for making jelly or fluid mounts, and for cementing cells and coverglasses to slides. In routine work, where large numbers of resin-mounted preparations are made and examined, square coverglasses are used for economy. The art of ringing a finished preparation is traditionally the preserve of the skilled amateur microscopist, yet where a preparation must be sealed properly, circular coverglasses and the ringing table are essential. Using a ringing table confers the advantage of applying multiple rings neatly, in a manner not possible by freehand.

A ring of shellac cement (usually made up in ethanol) serves to hold the coverglass in place where the mountant remains fluid or sets slowly. Enamel modeller's paint can also be used, and slides can be colour-coded as desired. Cements serve to exclude oxygen from resin-mounted preparations, prevent later crazing, and reduce fading of stains. This is particularly true for naturally derived resinous mountants, such as Canada balsam. Where the mountant is made up in the same solvent as the ringing shellac (usually ethanol), a barrier ring of cement in a different solvent must first be applied to prevent the shellac diffusing into the preparation, and causing a faint brown tint to colour the whole area.

7.10.1 Using a ringing table

A turned brass table (*Figure 7.2*) rotates upon a steel ball bearing held in the hollow at the top of the mild steel spindle, which forms the base plate. The turntable has concentric rings engraved upon its surface to assist in centering the slide, which is crucial. The base has been made from close-grained hardwood; the example has deliberately been lengthened to provide support for the forearm, but this is a matter of preference. The slide is held in position with two spring clips from an old microscope stage. A slightly different design has been published by Gerakaris (1984), or ringing tables can be purchased commercially.

The shape of the brush and the consistency of the ringing cement is of great importance to ensure a neat and clean result. If the cement is too thin, it will not provide an adequate seal, and is liable to run laterally on application; if too thick the ring will be uneven. To prepare a suitable brush, take a 00 artist's sable brush, hold back the hairs, and allow contact adhesive to permeate most of the brush down to the ferrule. Wipe the hairs back into place quickly with the fingers, and the brush will set. The top half of the bristle is left clean and cut as in *Figure 7.3*. In this way the brush does not splay on application, resulting in a thin incomplete and messy ring. The flexible tip should be cleaned in ethanol after use, and a few drops of ethanol added to the shellac to keep it fluid.

The centre of the position that the cell or coverslip should occupy can be marked by drawing around the edges of the slide onto paper and

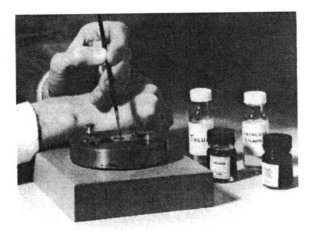

Figure 7.2: The ringing table.

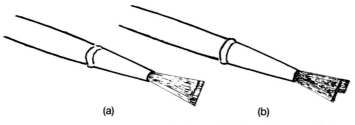

(a)   (b)

Figure 7.3: The ringing brush. The brush is glued rigid near the ferrule, as described in the text. It should then be wiped flat to form a chisel edge, which is then chamfered (using a tile support) on both sides with a razor (a). Ensure that the few hairs at the very tip remain free of glue. In use the brush should not be cleaned with solvent, but excess shellac wiped off with dry tissue. When next used, dip first into solvent to render the brush pliable. The size of the ring can be determined by altering the angle of the brush. After frequent use the chisel edge tends to assume the shape seen in (b). (I am grateful to Mr K.-D. Kemp, for permission to quote this description).

constructing the diagonals. Other positions can be computed as required. Place the slide upside down on the jig; mark the centre with India ink or marker pen (or transfer a circle of the diameter required if the table has no centre). Re-insert the slide the correct way up, centre it, and set the table spinning. It is easy to see if the slide is off-centre. Repeat this procedure until satisfied that the slide is central.

Charge the brush with the solvent and then sufficiently thinned sealant or varnish. Have some blotting paper handy to take off any gross excess from the brush. The idea is not to paint the ring on: this results in a wide, and often uneven ring which reflects the pressure used to paint it. Rather, allow the varnish to flow off the brush onto the slide, to give a ring which stands slightly proud and seals the edge of the coverslip. This knack comes quickly with practice.

Some people prefer to 'knife' the ringing seal on the coverslip to provide a very thin aesthetic border to the preparation. The wet seal is taken off the edge of the coverslip to provide the merest seal. Most workers prefer to construct a thicker seal which flows over the coverslip edge in a wave as it is applied, and affords greater protection to the preparation.

7.10.2 Labelling

Those slides which need to be labelled while being stained can be marked with an indelible pen or soft pencil, either on a white border or a frosted glass end. The classical alternative is to use a diamond pencil, but this lacks contrast, and may not always be so easy to use. For later reference it is best to use gummed sticky-backed labels. These can be bought with the name of an individual or institute on them, or printed out using a suitable computer programme.

Alternatively, one can use a fine draughtsman's pen to write the label (e.g. Rotring pen), as in *Figure 7.4*. The pen has a 0.2 mm nib for the fine, and 0.3 mm nib for the bolder type. Black Rotring ink was employed which is resistant to alcohol, xylene and water. In addition to the name of the specimen, the fixative and stain(s) used should be noted (where this has been the case) and details of where the specimen or sample was collected.

7.10.3 Transport

The subject of transport can be a sensitive one. The Post Office give no guarantee of safety, and it is disappointing to receive broken goods. Several

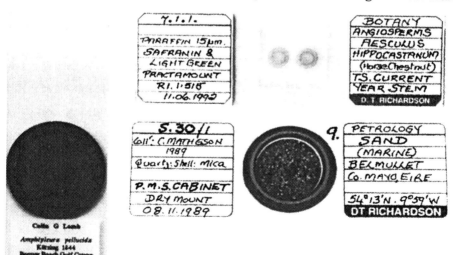

Figure 7.4:   Labelled slides, showing various forms and labels. (I am grateful to Mr D.T. Richardson and Mr C.G. Lamb for providing these slides).

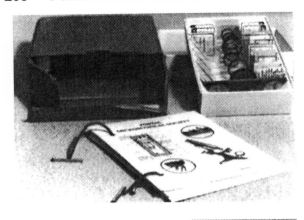

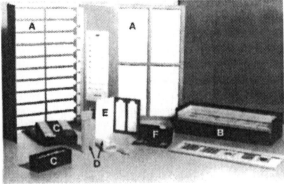

Figure 7.5: Transporting slides. The top illustration shows the corrugated cardboard box, designed by Mr D.T. Richardson, and notebook used by the Postal Microscopical Society. The notebook slides under the expanded polystyrene strips, which together prevent movement of the cardboard slide holder shown to the right of the picture. The bottom illustration shows a selection of alternative transport and storage methods. The two large slide trays (A) will accommodate up to 20, and the small slide tray (B) eight 3" × 1" slides each. Two examples of slide boxes (C) are shown front left. Four types of slide mailer are shown in the centre (D–F). The plastic slide mailers (D) will hold two to four slides, and are commonly used by cytological laboratory services. A card double-slide mailer (E) and a rigid plastic type (F) are also shown (with permission from the Postal Microscopical Society).

types of commercially available mailer are shown in *Figure 7.5*. The plastic types are usually more rigid than the individual cardboard mailers, which can bend along their long axis—a few millimetres is all that is needed to ruin the preparation. A rigid plastic box with individual partitions is the best of all. If such a box is used, it is advisable to pack any internal movement within the slots by using tissue paper or foam sheet.

The outer design of corrugated-card box used by the Postal Microscopical Society in conjunction with a cardboard 12-slide box permits room for a notebook, and is robust. The internal protection is made from expanded polystyrene, and the entire weight is about 50 g.

7.11 Artifacts

This section has been included at the end of the book, not to leave the reader discouraged, but rather to impress the statement made at the begining that all preparations of once-living material are artifactual. These artifacts are often determined by the manner in which the material is prepared, and this must be kept in mind when interpreting the final result. Artifacts are either the distortion or the loss of existing structural morphology; the displacement or the loss of diffusible substances; or the addition of material not present in the living state. The art of good specimen preparation is to prepare a neat slide in a simple manner, with the minimum of artifacts. In biological specimen preparation, *the least treatment is the best treatment.* For example, the usual preparation is made after hardening in a protein denaturant for some hours, when the tissues are thoroughly dehydrated with solvent extraction of lipids. They are then cooked at 60°C for some time, immobilized, shattered and compressed on a sharp edge, and the tissue slice stretched to its limits by surface tension. The tissue is further heated and dried before being washed, coloured and glued between two pieces of glass. We must expect artifacts in such cases!

A very comprehensive review of artifacts in thin tissue sections has been published by Wallington (1979) and Thompson and Luna (1978), to which the reader is referred for greater detail. A list of contaminants and artifacts commonly found in cytology specimens has been written by Proctor (1989). Tissues are naturally soft before fixation, and susceptible to mechanical damage; care should be taken in dissection and excision. Crushed nuclei and re-orientated (parallel) connective tissue fibres are common in poorly handled tissues, and serrated-tooth forceps should not be used. The cytoplasm of populations of single cells is particularly prone to mechanical damage from sampling, resulting in bare nuclei, or those whose cytoplasm has altered staining characteristics. Lubricating fluid (which gives rise to vacuolated areas in the smear with cells around the periphery) and fibres are possible contaminants arising from poor collecting technique.

Severe shrinkage will occur in those tissues which have been allowed to dry out before being fixed; equally serious during dissection is the introduction of contaminants, often starch powder from disposable gloves, or cork, wood or pitch from the surfaces of dissection boards. Starch particles are birefringent, showing the 'Maltese Cross of polarization', and weakly eosinophillic. Other major pre-fixation artifacts include autolysis (with loss of cell components, organ morphology and a uniform purple staining from H & E) and ice-crystal damage from samples which have been frozen too slowly prior to frozen sectioning.

Inadequate fixation will inevitably lead to inadequate processing and sectioning, with severe distortion and shrinkage of tissue. Even with adequate fixation, some distortion will occur, but this can be ameliorated to some extent by embedding in celloidin or resin rather than wax; another approach is to use secondary fixatives. The distortion caused by sectioning can be reduced, if unacceptable, by cutting thinner sections. A common example of gross changes in tissue structure occurring during fixation has been documented by Fox *et al.* (1985). Where short (2–4 h) fixation times in 10% formalin are followed by subsequent dehydration in ethyl alcohol, the fixation image may reflect that given by alcohol rather than formaldehyde, since the effect of the 10% formalin may be reversed by partial washing out and replacement by the alcohol. This phenomenon is more likely to occur on an automatic processor left on an overnight cycle than when fixation and subsequent dehydration is monitored by the worker.

Old fixatives can cause contamination, either from extraneous tissues or from the production of pigments. Prolonged fixation can cause lack of nuclear staining; whether substances are translocated within tissues will depend very much on the rate of penetration of the fixative mixture compared to its primary constituents, or the solubility of cell components. Glycogen streaming, following alcohol fixation, is a well-known example. Vacuoles left in fatty tissues where lipids have been dissolved and lost are another.

Perfusion fixation has its own peculiar associated artifacts. A good perfusion is only possible if the vasculature has been well washed to avoid the formation of thrombi. More rarely seen, but possible, is the translocation of cells or tissue fragments between specimens. This is particularly so in cytology where exfoliated cells (floaters) may be transferred from one specimen to another during dehydration through the alcohol series, or whilst staining. Translocation of tissue fragments is also possible during processing, where friable tissues should be wrapped in close-weave, lint-free gauze. The water used for floating out sections should also be changed frequently for the same reason.

Further artifacts occur during tissue processing subsequent to fixation. The decalcification of bone to permit sectioning is an example of an artifact introduced intentionally. However, initial sawing of the bone may cause splintering or deposition of bone debris with associated nuclear crushing or connective tissue translocation. Acid decalcifiers, although fast, cause more tissue artifacts than slower-acting decalcifiers such as 10% formic acid and EDTA.

Ice-crystal artifact and vacuolation have been mentioned; other examples of structural damage are the appearance of regular pinholes caused by gas evolution, as well as the fissures seen in tissues exposed to hardening fixatives and rapid solvent evaporation during dehydration and clearing. These are often seen in the liver and spleen, and are more common in wax- than plastic-embedded tissues.

The often drastic effects of tissue shrinkage artifacts caused by dehydration and impregnation by hot embeddding media may have serious implications for morphometric studies. A certain amount of further distortion caused by compression during microtomy is inevitable—although this can be counteracted by stretching (itself an artifact) the section. Nevertheless, most of the artifacts that may be introduced during microtomy are easily recognized and avoided by using well-sharpened knives and careful technique. *Tables 4.1* and *4.2* deal with fault finding in microtomy and how to recognize and avoid scores, tears, chattering and undue compression. Two other artifacts that are avoidable are: firstly, the embedding of dust and grit from dirty bench surfaces where blocks have been placed face down prior to cutting; and secondly, tearing and disruption of the faced block after severe rough-cutting.

Picking up the section and mounting, either from the water-bath, or onto hot adhesive on the slide, can leave wrinkles or stretch the section. If the section is then blotted, care must be taken not to ruin the tissue, and soft sections, such as brain, should only be blotted when it is likely that they will not adhere well to the slide. Sections left too long in a water-bath can stain poorly and collagen components can swell in disproportion to the rest of the section thickness. Likewise, soluble components can leach out of the section (which has a high surface area) at this stage. Incomplete removal of wax or resin embedding medium can lead to retention of wax and inferior staining (Nedzel, 1951). GMA sections that have been stained with H & E have shown folds and cracking in tissue-free areas; this has been shown to be due to very pure samples of GMA lacking cross-linking impurities (Gerrits and Suurmeijer, 1991).

Most staining is by diffusion, and since artifacts are largely caused by mechanical and chemical effects, few artifacts are caused as a direct result of staining. The most common artifacts are caused by variations in section thickness, and the use of old solutions or batches of dye. Due to the work of the Biological Stains Commission, faulty dye samples are rare. However, most stains are prone to fading—particularly if they have been badly cleared, mounted in acidic mounting media or exposed to sunlight.

Specimens are susceptible to mechanical damage inflicted during mounting and finishing of the preparation. A coverglass which has been forcefully applied may disrupt the section or whole mount, and bubbles may remain in the mountant. Sections which are allowed to dry out before mountant is applied may have air bubbles trapped in the protoplasm, which appears as a 'deposit'. Dry mounts that have been incompletely dessicated may support the growth of micro-organisms, while fluid mounts that have been less than meticulously sealed will, sooner or later, leak.

7.12 Restoring preparations

7.12.1 Repairing broken slides

The major disadvantage of glass slides is that they are prone to breakage. Where the specimen has been mounted onto the coverglass, and this has been left intact, then it can be soaked off in xylene, or water if an aqueous mountant, and remounted onto a fresh slide.

More usually the section has been mounted onto the slide, which has then been broken. Merely cementing a support slide onto the underside of the various bits assembled like a jigsaw puzzle will serve to double the thickness of the glass, and prevent the condenser being used properly but, if the specimen is valuable, it is often better than nothing!

The coverglass should be soaked off in xylene, and the section covered in a thin layer of DPX. This should be allowed to set and the slide chilled. The section can then be stripped from the slide, the DPX dissolved away and the section mounted onto a fresh slide using a 'hockey stick'. An alternative method is to substitute a 1:6 mixture of DPX to butyl acetate for the DPX above. The resin is painted on in the same way, and left on a hot-plate or in an incubator at 40°C to dry for 30 min. After drying, the resin is cut with a sharp scalpel blade, and the section floated off onto distilled water. The section is transferred onto the new slide, dried on the hot-plate, washed in several changes of butyl acetate, then in xylene and re-mounted.

7.12.2 Restaining faded sections

Remove the coverslip by placing the section into a Coplin jar containing xylene, in a fume hood, for as long as necessary to allow the coverglass to fall off: about half an hour should be sufficient. Do not be persuaded to slide the coverglass off the slide, as this can damage the preparation. Rehydrate the section through the alcohols to 70% ethanol. Remove excess stain by washing for 10 min in 10% hydrochloric acid in 70% alcohol. Alteratively, use 5% ammonia in 70% alcohol.

Excess stain may also be removed at this stage by bleaching. Bring the section to distilled water (instead of using acid alcohol). Flood the slide with 0.25% potassium permanganate for 5 min. Wash with tap water, and bleach the section with 1% oxalic acid. For both methods, wash thoroughly in tap, followed by distilled, water.

7.12.3 Restoring tissues dried during processing

Once immersed in transition medium, or aqueous solutions for processing, tissues or sections should not be allowed to dry. Should this be the case, the following protocol may give partial success (Bancroft and Stevens, 1990). Transfer the tissues to a sealed vessel containing the following.

70% ethyl alcohol	70 ml
Glycerol	30 ml
Dithionite	1 g

Leave in the solution overnight, or for several hours minimum. Recommence tissue processing at the dehydration stage in the normal way. Use an adhesive to mount the sections of such damaged tissues. Smears which have been air-dried may be re-hydrated in 0.9% sodium chloride for 30 sec and fixed in 95% ethanol, before proceeding.

For re-swelling dried arthropods the following procedure can be used (Gray, 1954).

Distilled water	30 ml
Acetic acid	30 ml
Chloral hydrate	40 ml

For dried-out dried plant tissue use the following.

Distilled water	25 ml
Lactic acid	50 ml
95% ethyl alcohol	25 ml

Soak the specimens in the mixture for a few hours, depending upon the thickness and hardness of the tissue. Resume the processing of the arthropods, after washing gently in distilled water. Botanical material should be washed gently in 50% ethanol before proceeding as before.

References

Aumonier FJ, Setterington R. (1967) Some notes on the mounting of histological sections. *Proc. R. Microscop. Soc.* **2**, 428–429.

Bancroft JD, Cook HC. (1984) *Manual of Histological Techniques.* Churchill Livingstone, Edinburgh.

Bancroft JD, Stevens A. (eds) 1990) *Theory and Practice of Histological Techniques*, 3rd edn. Churchill Livingstone, Edinburgh.

Barr WT. (1970) Effects of sunlight on stained sections mounted in various media. *Stain Technol.* **45**, 9–14.

Bissing DR. (1974) Haupt's gelatin adhesive mixed with formalin for affixing paraffin sections to slides. *Stain Technol.* **49**, 116–117.

Bradbury S. (1969) A commercial guage suitable for the measurement of coverglass thickness. *J. Quekett Microscop. Club* **31**, 214–216.

Bradbury S. (1973) *Peacock's Elementary Microtechnique*, 4th revised edn. Edward Arnold, London.

Fink S. (1978a) Some new methods for affixing sections to glass slides. I. Aqueous adhesives. *Stain Technol.* **62**, 27–33.

Fink S. (1978b) Some new methods for affixing sections to glass slides. II. Organic-solvent based adhesives. *Stain Technol.* **62**, 93–99.

Fink S. (1978c) Some new methods for affixing sections to glass slides. III. Pressure-sensitive adhesives. *Stain Technol.* **62**, 349–354.

Fox CH, Johnson FB, Whiting J, Roller PP. (1985) Formaldehyde fixation. *J. Histochem. Cytochem.* **33**, 845–853.

Franklin AL, Fillion WG. (1985) A new technique for retarding fading of fluorescence: DPX-BME. *Stain Technol.* **60**, 125–135.

Gerakaris JG. (1984) Slide ringing re-visited. *Microscope* **32**, 259–264.

Gerrits PO, Suurmeijer AJH. (1991) Glycol methacrylate embedding in diagnostic pathology. *Am. J. Clin. Pathol.* **95**, 150–156.

Gray P. (1954) *The Microtomist's Formulary and Guide.* Blakiston, New York.

Hollander DH, Frost JK. (1970) Annual bands in synthetic-resin-mounted microscopic slides. *Acta Cytol.* **14**, 142–144.

Hollander DH, Frost JK. (1971) Antioxidant inhibition of stain fading and mounting medium crazing. *Acta Cytol.* **15**, 419.

Humason GL. (1972) *Animal Tissue Techniques,* 3rd edn. WH Freeman, San Francisco, CA.

Johnson GD, Nogueira Araujo G MdeC. (1981) A simple method of reducing the fading of immunofluorescence during microscopy. *J. Immunol. Methods* **43**, 349–350.

Johnson GD, Davidson RS, McNamee KC, Russell G, Goodwin D, Holbarrow J. (1982) Fading of immunofluorescence during microscopy: a study of the phenomenon and its remedy. *J. Immunol. Methods* **55**, 231–242.

Lillie RD, Windle WF, Zirkle C. (1950) Interim report of the committee on histologic mounting media: resinous media. *Stain Technol.* **25**, 1–9.

Lillie RD, Zirkle C, Greco JP. (1953) Final report of the committee on histologic mounting media. *Stain Technol.* **28**, 57–80.

Nedzel GA. (1951) Intranuclear birefringent inclusions—an artifact occuring in paraffin sections. *Q. J. Microscop. Sci.* **92**, 343–346.

Pluta M. (1988) *Advanced Light Microscopy Vol. 1. Principles and Basic Properties.* Elsevier, Amsterdam.

Proctor DT. (1989) Staining techniques. In *Clinical Cytotechnology.* (eds DV Coleman and PA Chapman). Butterworths, London, pp. 75–105.

Rawlins DJ (1992) *Light Microscopy.* BIOS Scientific Publishers Ltd, Oxford.

Schmolke C. (1993) Effects of mounting media on fading of Toluidine Blue and Pyronin G staining in epoxy sections. *Biotechnic Histochem.* **68**, 132–136.

Setterington R. (1953) The specifications of a standard microscope cover-glass. *J. R. Microscop. Soc.* **73**, 69–76.

Silverman M. (1986) Light-polymerizing plastics as slide mounting media. *Stain Technol.* **61**, 135–136.

Spinnell BM, Loveland RP. (1960) Optics of the object space in microscopy. *J. Microsc.* **79**, 59–80.

Thompson SW, Luna L. (1978) *An Atlas of Artifacts Encountered in the Preparation of Microscopic Tissue Sections.* Thomas, Springfield.

Thornton J, Hendrickson B, Harralson C. (1985) Tolerance and uniformity of microscope coverslips. *Microscope* **33**, 179–185.

Valnes K, Brandtzaeg P. (1985) Retardation of immunofluorescence fading during microscopy. *J. Histochem. Cytochem.* **33**, 755–361.

Wallington EA. (1979) Artifacts in tissue sections. *Med. Lab. Sci.* **36**, 3–61.

White GW. (1974) The correction of tubelength to compensate for coverglass thickness variations. *Microscopy* **32**, 411–420.

Woolfe G. (1983) The importance of cover-slip thickness. *Microscopy* **34**, 604–607.

Appendix A
Safety

Most of the reagents used to prepare biological specimens for microscopy are toxic, carcinogenic and dangerous to use. They should be handled with care and stored safely. This appendix gives an outline only of the major hazards. The principal routes into the body are by inhalation, ingestion and by skin contact. Risks are increased with hot or volatile reagents. All containers for liquids (Winchesters, litre bottles) should be carried in suitably designed carriers, and never by the neck of the bottle.

The COSHH regulations are legally binding, and provide for the safe handling, storage and disposal of a large number of potentially hazardous chemicals; reliance is also placed on observing the principles of Good Laboratory Practice. Risk assessments should be made regularly, and contingency plans should be in place to deal with emergencies; for further details see Tawney (1992), Howl (1986) and the World Health Organisation *Laboratory Biosafety Manual* (1983). A good series of safety articles has recently been published (Orton, 1993), which although specifically written for schools, is nevertheless useful for other workers.

Maximum exposure limits (threshold limit values) provide a quantitative assessment of the risk by inhalation, and these are given below. Ingestion should be a negligible risk, since smoking, drinking and eating should *never* take place in the laboratory under any circumstances. Chemical contact with skin and clothes can be reduced by having suitable gloves, coats and masks available. Polythene disposable gloves are the most resistant to resins and liquid chemicals. Take extra care when using organic solvents such as xylene and acetone, and use forceps to handle slides and specimens. Eye goggles should be worn where there is a risk of splashing from a vigorous reaction, and an eye-wash bottle and first-aid kit should be kept in the laboratory. Personal coats and bags should be kept outside the laboratory, and hand-washing facilities should be located inside the laboratory for use before leaving.

Fixatives

Most fixatives are toxic, volatile, and may irritate the eyes and respiratory system. Fixatives should be disposed of by flushing to waste with copious (e.g. 50 × volume) amounts of water. Heavy metals and their fixatives should not be washed down the sink or incinerated, but should be precipitated out: see Lewis *et al.* (1983). Inactivate spilt fixatives using dried milk powder or commercial absorbent spillage packs. For precautions regarding formaldehyde see Ashford *et al.* (1983, 1984) and Salkie (1991). Enclosed tissue processors are now available to reduce leakage of fumes (Edwards and Campbell, 1984a, b).

Dehydration and transition (clearing) agents

Most of these chemicals are volatile and flammable (Maxwell, 1978). They should be stored in the smallest necessary volume in a flammable store, and used in a fume hood or well-ventilated part of the laboratory. Benzene and dioxan are rarely used because they are both carcinogenic and toxic. Ether and propylene dioxide are explosive in the presence of open flames. Flammable solvents should never be stored in a domestic refrigerator. There are derivatives from food-oils (e.g. Histoclear®) which have certain limited applications in place of xylene. Exposure of the eyes to organic solvents may cause conjunctivitis.

Embedding media

Nitrocellulose embedding involves the use of very flammable reagents. Ether is one of the most flammable laboratory reagents; fumes can be ignited by a naked flame over several metres, causing bottles of fluid to explode. Resins emit vapours and will form aerosols during polymerization, and the oven used should be vented to the outside. The monomers are flammable, and dry BPO is explosive. Waste resins should be polymerized for several days at 60°C before disposal in unbreakable bottles. All monomers should be mixed in disposable containers, and hands washed with soap and *cold* water after use. Resin blocks are never completely polymerized and should be sawn to size in a fume hood.

Stains and dyes

Most dyes are used as powders which are potentially teratogenic and carcinogenic. They should be weighed out and dissolved carefully. Skin contact during staining should be minimized. Strong acids should be diluted by addition to water, and not vice versa. Both dilute acids and alkalis can cause blindness if splashed in the eyes.

Carcinogens

(i)   All carcinogenic substances should be placed in a resealable bag contained in a locked cabinet, unless a refrigerator is indicated.
(ii) Gloves and a face-mask should be worn, and weighing should be carried out on a balance kept in a fume hood, lined with plastic-backed paper.
(iii) All glassware should be rinsed in cold water after use, and gloves and waste material sent for incineration.
(iv) Where skin contact results, wash for 10 min in copious cold water.

Biohazards

All tissue should be fixed before handling, but where this is not possible (in preparing cytological specimens) aerosols and splashes should be avoided; these can be created by opening specimen bottles, filling cytocentrifuges and pipetting. Phenolic disinfectants are used for organic material; hypochlorites and glutaraldehyde for viruses; and formalin vapour for cryostats and safety microbiological cabinets. Tuberculous material can be inactivated by fixation in hot (60°C) 10% formalin overnight. Instruments and biological material which are potentially infected with HIV or Hepatitis B may be sterilized by fixation in glutaraldehyde.

References

Ashford NA, Ryan WC, Caldart CC. (1983, 1984) Law and science policy in federal regulation of formaldehyde. *Science* **222**, 894–900; Letters. *Science* **224**, 550–556.
Barrow AJ. (1988) Laboratory Safety. *Inst. Med. Lab. Sci. Gazette* April, 203–208.

Causton BE, RMS Safety Sub-committee. (1981) Resins: toxicity, hazards and safe handling. *Proc. R. Microscop. Soc.* **16**, 265–271.

Department of Education and Science (1978) *Safety in Science Laboratories, 3rd edn.* HMSO, London.

Edwards FP, Campbell AR. (1984a) An enclosed fixative preparation system. *Med. Lab. Sci.* **41**, 285–287.

Edwards FP, Campbell AR. (1984b) The removal of formaldehyde and xylene fumes from histopathology laboratories: a functional approach to the design of extraction systems. *J. Clin. Pathol.* **37**, 401–408.

Howl AJ. (1986) Techniques of safety management in the laboratory. *Inst. Med. Lab. Sci. Gazette* February, 69–71.

Lewis PR, RMS Safety Committee. (1983) Fixatives: hazards and safe handling. *Proc. R. Microscop. Soc.* **18**, 164–169.

Maxwell MH. (1978) Safer substitutes for xylene and propylene oxide in histology, haematology, and electron microscopy. *Med. Lab. Sci.* **35**, 401–403.

Orton RJJ. (1993) Safety XII, the use of ionizing radiations and radioactive sources. *School Sci. Rev.* **74**, part 268, 7–16.

Salkie ML. (1991) The prevalence of atopy and hypersensitivity to formaldehyde in pathologists. *Arch. Pathol. Lab. Med.* **115**, 614–616.

Tawney D. (1992) Assessment of risk and school science. *School Sci. Rev.* **74**, part 267, 7–14.

World Health Organisation (1983) *Laboratory Safety Manual.* WHO, Geneva.

Appendix B
Refractive indices

Refractive indices of mountants and immersion media

	RI at 20°C
Mountants	
Apathy's gum syrup	1.52
Aquamount	1.38
Canada balsam, natural	1.52
Canada balsam, neutral in xylene	1.53
DPX (BDH/Merck)	1.52
DPX in xylene	1.53
Diaphane (neutral or green)	1.48
Dirax	1.65
Entellan (new)	1.49
Euparal	1.48
Euparal vert	1.52
Farrants' medium	1.42
Gelatin	1.41
Glycerin albumen (Mayer's)	1.42
Glycerol jelly	1.44–1.47
Gum arabic	1.42–1.51
Hyrax	1.71
Lacto-phenol	1.44
α-Monobromonaphthalene	1.66
Naphrax	1.69
Pleurax	1.75
Realgar	2.18
Sirax	1.81
XAM neutral medium	1.49
Immersion media	
Cedarwood oil	1.516
Ethyl alcohol	1.432
Ethylene glycol (Carbowax)	1.432
Glycerol	1.470

Refractive indices, *continued*

	RI at 20°C
Paraffin oil	1.480
Toluene	1.496
Water, distilled	1.333
Xylene	1.498
Commercial immersion oil	1.515
Biological	
Cell contents (fixed and cleared)	1.53–1.54
Cytoplasm, living	1.353
Diatom silica	1.430
Protein (dry)	1.540

Index

Abrasives, 106–107
Accelerators, 64, 65, 66, 69, 162
Accentuators, 162
Acetic acid, 17, 18, 19, 22
Acetone, 19, 21, 72
Acidophil tissue, 22, 75, 160–161
Acridine orange, 183–184
Acrolein, 19, 20–21
Acrylic resins, 64, 67–70, 76, 172–173, 199
Adhesives, 35, 54–55, 75, 142, 198–200
Agar, 57, 62–63, 144
Air bubbles, 194–195, 209
Alcian blue 8GX, 199
Alcohol fixatives, 13, 21, 22, 138–139
Allen's B-15, 13, 27
Amman's lacto-phenol, 30
Ante-medium, 39
    see also Transition media
Anti-coagulants, 15
Anti-oxidants, 193, 202
Anti-roll bar, 102–103
Anti-roll plate, 101, 102–103
Apathy's medium, 151, 154, 191
Aqueous mountants, 191–192
Araldite, 64–67
Artifacts, 1, 8, 11, 15, 23, 207–209
Autolysis, 11, 207
Automated microtomes, 89
Automatic
    schedules, 44–45
    staining, 177, 179
Auxochrome, 160

B-4, 24
B-5, 13, 24
B-15, 13, 27
Bacterial stains, 184–186
Baker's fluid, 124
Base-sledge microtomes, 87–88, 92–93
Basiphil tissue, 22, 160
Beilby layer, 94
Berlèse funnel, 4
Bevel angle, 90, 92, 93, 116
    see also Cutting angle
Biconcave knife, 90–91, 108
Biebrich scarlet, 167, 171

Biological Stain Commission, 188
Biopsies, 5, 137
Blayde's preservative, 29, 30
Bleaching, 77–78, 187, 193, 210
Block
    staining, 173
    trimming, 50–51, 99, 101, 127
Blueing, 165
Böhm–Sprenger's, 28
Bone, 68, 72–76, 91–92
Bouin's, 13, 27, 187
Brat's method, 171–172

Cambridge rocking microtome, 85–86
Canada balsam, 193, 201
Carbowax — see PEG waxes
Carmine, 166, 173
Carnoy's, 13, 27, 42, 43, 78, 177
Carnoy–Lebrun's, 13, 27
Cavity slides, 2, 151, 152
Cedarwood oil, 42–43, 47, 61, 193
Celestine blue, 164
Cell
    adherence, 141–142
    blocks, 144
    loss, 8–9, 141–142
    monolayers, 28, 62
Celloidin, 60, 118, 132, 169, 182, 193, 198, 200
Cellulose sections, 41, 60–62, 118, 123
    see also LVN
Champy's, 13, 26
Chemical dehydration, 41–42
Chitin, 21, 78–79
Chloroform, 42
Chrome-acetic, 25
Chromic acid, 19, 21–22
Chromium trioxide — see chromic acid
Chromo-acetic-formalin — see CRAF
Chromophore, 159–160
Chucks, 89–90, 96
Clamps — see chucks
Clarke's, 13, 28, 42
Cleaning slides, 200–201
Clearance angle, 96, 109, 110, 116, 117, 125

Clearing, 77–78, 151
Clearing agents, 39
  see also Transition media
Coated slides, 58, 198–200
Coated tissue, 17
Collecting material, 3–5, 137–138
Collection records, 4–5, 205
Columbia jar, 197
Compression, 113–116
Control tissues, 188
Counterstains, 166–167
Counting cells, 183–184
Coverslip thickness, 195–197
Coverslip thickness correction, 196
CRAF, 13, 25, 76
Crazing, 201–202
Cryogenic fluids, 99–100
Cryostats, 96, 97, 98, 123
  disinfecting, 101
  sectioning, 26, 27, 101–105, 120, 123,
    128–130
Cryotomy, 27, 96–97, 120, 128–130
  temperatures, 102
  trimming, 101
Cutting
  angle, 88, 90, 91, 92, 93, 96, 105, 112,
    115, 125
  speed, 117–118, 119, 120, 125
Cytocentrifugation, 1, 139–140
Cytological
  fixation, 13, 137–139
  stains, 174–179

de Castro's fluid, 73
Decalcification, 23, 24, 68, 73–76, 208
Decalcifying agents, 73–74
Defatting, 71, 76
Dehydration, 39, 41–42, 56, 67, 69, 71,
    121–122, 150, 169, 192–193, 208
  chemical, 41–42
Detachment of sections, 199–200
DGD, 59–60
Diatom frustules, 79–80
Dichromate–sulphuric, 200–201
Differentiation, 70, 161, 163, 165, 174,
    175, 178, 180, 182, 183, 184, 185
Digoxygenin, 165–166
Dioxan, 43, 63
Displacement, 162
Disposable blades, 94–95, 101
Dissection, 15
Distortion, 20, 93, 113–116, 207–208
Double embedding, 61–62, 78
Double-pass microtomes, 86
DPX, 144, 172–173, 193–194, 201, 202, 210
Dry
  ice, 97
  mounts, 2, 147, 148–150
Drying agents, 41, 150

Dyes
  amphoteric, 160–161, 174, 177
  definition of, 159
  nomenclature, 159–160
  purity, 187–188
  standardization, 187–188

EDTA, 73, 74
Elder pith, 96, 132
Electron microscope, 7
  techniques, 5, 7, 13, 15, 18, 64, 71
Electrostatic charges, 24, 102–103,
    124–125
Elftman's, 26
Embedding
  centres, 48
  media, 39, 46
  media, gelatin, 57, 62
  tissues, 46–48, 122
End-point determination, 74–75
Eosin, 167
Eosin-azure, 177–178
Epon, 65, 66
Epoxy resins, 65–67
Erythrocytes, 3
  lysing fluids, 137
Essential oils, 43
Ester wax, 59
Ethanol, 13, 17
Ether-alcohol, 13, 28
Euparal, 194, 201

FAA, 13, 24, 30, 76
Facet, 93–94, 107–109
  angle, 91, 92–94
  polish, 94, 105, 109, 112
Fading, 29, 171, 192, 193, 201–203,
    209–210
Farrants' medium, 151, 154, 192
Fibres, 79
Field fixative, 27
Field's stain, 174
Fixation
  absence, 17
  function, 1, 11, 14, 120–121, 125
  immersion, 14–15, 207
  perfusion, 15–16, 208
  phase-partition, 16, 28
Fixatives
  osmolarity, 18, 121, 155
  pH, 18, 21
  primary, 19–22
  see also under name of formulator
Fixed tissues, storage, 58
Flemming without acetic — *see* FWA
Flemming's, 13, 26, 29
Flexibilizers, 65
'Floaters', 138–139, 178
Floc, 80, 183

Fluid mounts, 1, 2, 147, 151–153, 154, 157
Fluorochromes, 183–184, 202
FNAB, 137
Folds, 53, 54, 55, 65, 66, 70, 102, 209
Foster and Gifford's fluid, 124
Foraminifera, 149–150
Formaldehyde, 19–20, 35
Formalin, 13, 18, 19–20, 23, 29, 35, 58,
   101, 177, 186
  advantages, 20
  pigment, 20, 186
Formalin-alcohol, 13, 23
Formic acid, 73, 74
Formol-acetic-alcohol — see FAA
Formol-calcium, 13, 23, 96
Formol-saline, 13, 23, 29
Formol-sublimate, 13, 24
Formol-sucrose, 13, 23
Formvar, 199
Free-floating staining, 97, 104, 119, 169,
   171, 193
Freehand sectioning, 131–133
Freeze
  drying, 17
  substitution, 17
Freezing
  damage, 97–99, 207–208
  microtome, 88–89
Frozen sections, 26, 27, 75, 96–105, 111,
   119, 123
  handling, 104
Frozen tissue, 58, 111
FWA, 26

Gatenby and Painter's preservative, 30
Gelatin-coated slides, 35, 198, 200
Gelvatol, 202
Gendre's, 13, 27
Giemsa stain, 172, 173, 174, 176–177
Glass slides, standard, 1
Gloves, 65, 207
Glutaraldehyde, 13, 19, 20–21, 57
Glycerol, 202
  jelly mounts, 1, 30, 148, 151, 154–157,
   171–172, 192
  mountant, 148, 151, 157
GMA, 64, 67–70, 72, 76, 92, 119, 123,
   172–173, 209
Gold-size, 30, 148, 149, 150, 152, 153
Gram reaction, 162, 184–186
Gum tragacanth, 149, 150
Gum media, 154–157

H & E, 170
H & E-phloxine, 172
Haematal 8, 164, 171, 173, 187
Haematoxylin and eosin — see H & E
Haematin pigment, 20, 186

Haematoxylin stains, 161–162, 163–165,
   170–171
Hair fibres, 79
Hand microtome, 85, 131–133
Handles, 90, 107–108
Hard tissues, 41, 52, 60, 64, 67, 68, 72–80,
   86, 91–92, 111, 114, 123, 131–132
Haupt's gelatin, 57, 198
Heating stains and fixatives, 17, 35, 168,
   186
Heidenhain's 'Azan', 182–183
Heidenhain's SUSA, 13, 21, 25, 187
Heiffor knife , 86, 90–91, 108
Helly's, 13, 21, 24, 29, 177, 187
  see also Zenker-formol
HEMA, 67
  see also GMA
Heterogenous tissues, 43, 60, 114
Historical development, 2
'Hockey stick', 119, 210
Holders — see Chucks
Hones, 106, 108–109
Honing, 105, 106–109
Hot-plate method, 54–55
Hydrochloric acid, 19, 73, 74
Hydrogen peroxide, 187
Hydrophilic
  resins, 63, 64, 70–71
  waxes, 59–60

Ice crystals, 97–99, 208
Immunocytochemistry, 2, 17, 20, 21, 35,
   58–59, 63, 64, 65, 67, 70, 71–72, 74,
   104, 173
Imprints, 1, 142–144
IMS, 41
In situ hybridization, 21, 166
Insect tissues, 78–79
Irrigation, 146–147, 183
Iso-electric point, 160

Janus green B, 184
Jeffrey's fluid, 146
Jenner's stain, 174, 176
Johansen's quadruple stain, 179, 180–182
Jung knife, 90

Kemet plate, 109
Kernechtrot, 165–166
Knife
  angles, 92–93, 125
  backs, 91, 107–108
  breakers, 95
  nicks, 106
  profiles, 90–92
  quality, 85, 125
  temper, 91, 106
Knives

care, 75, 85, 94, 97, 111
cold, 96–97
diamond, 96
etching, 94
glass, 95–96
polishing, 109
sharpening, 105–111, 125
types, 90–92

'L' pieces — see Leuckhart pieces
Labelling, 55, 205
Lactic acid, 30, 74
Lakes, 161–162
Lapping, 109
Leiden fixative, 34
Leishman's stain, 174, 176
Lendrum's,
   fixative, 24
   softening fluid, 124
Leuckhart pieces, 46, 50, 90
Leuco-
   bases, 162
   dyes, 162
Lewitsky–Baker's, 13, 24, 26
Light microscope, 5, 6, 8, 168
   techniques, 5, 6, 8–9, 79
Light polymerizing media, 194
Lignified tissues, 76–78
Lipids, 16–17, 26, 28, 41, 99, 144, 161
Liquid nitrogen, 58, 99–100
Lithium carbonate, 187
London resins, 42, 70–72
   see also LR White and LR Gold
Lowicryl resins, 70–71
LR Gold, 42, 71
LR White, 42, 70–72, 76, 199
Lubricants, 106–107
Lugol's iodine, 185, 187
LVN, 41, 60–62, 118, 123, 132, 169, 182,
   193, 198, 200
Lysochromes, 161, 162

Maceration, 2, 77, 78, 145–146
Macrotomes, 131
Malarial pigment, 186
Mallory's trichrome, 179–180
Manual
   processing, 40, 43–44
   sharpening, 108–111, 112
Marking slides, 55
Maximow's, 24
May-Grünwald, 174, 176
Mayer's albumen, 54, 55, 198
Mercuric chloride, 19, 21, 29
Mercuric chloride-formalin, 24
Mercury pigment, 187
Metachromasia, 162–163, 174
Metallic impregnation, 162, 173
Methacarn, 28, 42

Microwaves, 30–35, 150
   cryostat sections, 34, 104
   paraffin sections, 34
   processing, 32–34, 71, 144
   stains, 35
Minot microtome, 86
MMA, 67–68, 76, 92, 123
Mordants, 161–162, 163, 165, 167, 184–185
Mountant thickness, 197
Mountants, 14, 191–195
Mounting sections, 52–55
Mukerji's fluid, 78
Multi-spot slides, 63, 173
Multi-tissue blocks, 63
Multiple staining, 173–174

Nail varnish, 144
Naples clamp, 89
Navashin's, 13, 25
Negative staining, 162
Neutral stains, 174–179
Newcomer's, 13, 28
Nigrosin WS, 184
Nitric acid, 73, 74, 94, 200
Nitrocellulose, 60–62
   disadvantages, 62
Nitrogen, 71
   see also Liquid nitrogen
Nuclear fast red, 165–166
Nuclear stains, 163–166
Numerical aperture, 196, 197

Orange G, 177, 178
Osmium dioxide, 187
Osmium tetroxide, 18, 22, 187
Oversight stains, 65, 166, 170, 172,

Papanicolaou staining, 138–139, 160–161,
   164, 177–179
Paper moulds, 46, 48–50,
Paper-clip holders, 195
Paraffin wax, disadvantages, 63–64
Paraformaldehyde, 19, 20, 21, 23
Pectin–agar–sucrose, 57
PEG waxes, 34, 58–59, 138, 198
Peltier effect, 88
Pereyeni's fluid, 73
Perfusion chambers, 146–147, 148, 183
Periodate-lysine-paraformaldehyde —
   see PLD
Peterfi's method, 61, 78
Phagocytosis, 162
Phase-partition, 16–17, 28, 42–43
Phenol-formaldehyde, 20
Picric acid, 18, 19, 22, 74, 94, 186, 187
Pigments, 21–22, 186–187
Plasticizers, 65
PLP, 20
Polyethylene glycol — see PEG waxes

Poly-L-lysine-coated slides, 58
Polychrome stains, 179–183
Polyester waxes, 59–60
Polyvinyl alcohol–PEG embedding media, 58
Portable microscopes, 5
Post-fixation treatment, 29–30, 31, 32, 42, 99, 104, 132–133, 186–187
Postal Microscopical Society, 206
Potassium dichromate, 19, 21–22, 25, 161, 201
Pre-polymerization, 69–70
Preparations
  factors influencing, 3, 8–9, 12, 120–123, 138, 207–209
  interpreting, 8–9, 138
  studying, 8
  types, 1, 2
Preservatives, 14, 29, 137, 153, 192
Primary fixatives, 19
Processing
  cassettes, 21, 40
  recording, 80
  schedules, 43–45, 120–123
Progressive stains, 164

R-G stains, 138, 174–177, 202
Rake angle, 91, 92, 93, 113, 116, 125
Ralph knife, 75, 95–96, 123
Randolph's CRAF, 13, 25, 76
Rapid fixation, 27, 28, 43
Recording details, 4–5, 8, 80, 205
Refractive index — see RI
Refractory tissues, 52, 77, 124, 131
Régaud's, 13, 26
Regressive stains, 163
Rehydrating
  sections, 56
  tissues, 210–211
Repairing preparations, 209–211
Replicas, 142–144
Resin
  embedding media, 46, 63–72, 76, 77, 123
  mountant, 2, 147, 193–194
  removal, 72
Resins
  curing, 66
  sectioning, 70, 118–119
  staining, 65, 70, 172–173
Restaining sections, 210
Reuter's cement, 156
RI, 39, 151, 191, 217–218
Ribboning faults, 52
Ribbons, 24, 50, 51–52, 63, 92, 102, 115
  storing, 52
Richardson's stain, 172
Ringing
  brush, 203–204
  table, 148, 203–205

Rings for cells, 148–149, 152–153
Rossman's, 13, 27
Rotary microtomes, 86–87

Safety, 213–216
  cryogens, 99–100
  disinfecting, 101
  freezing, 99–100
  knives, 94
  microwaves, 35
  resins, 65
Safranin, 166
Salt-Zenker's, 25
Sanfelice's, 13, 25
Schaudinn's, 13, 28
Schultze's fluid, 145
Scott's tap water substitute, 165
Secondary fixation, 29
Section thickness, 46, 63–64, 85–87, 95–96, 99, 111, 117, 119–120, 132
Sectioning, 111–112, 116–120, 125, 126–130, 131–133
  faults, 120, 123, 126–130
  freehand, 131–133
  speed, 117–119, 120, 125
Sections
  hardening, 199
  lifting, 24, 28, 75, 199–200
  locating, 55
Sedimentation, 139–141
Serial sections, 2, 52, 53, 63, 70, 87–88, 96, 102, 118
Sharpening
  machines, 105
  stones, 108
Silane-coated slides, 58, 198–199
Simple fixatives, 19
Single-pass microtomes, 86
Sintered knives, 91–92
Size, tissue processing, 120–123
Slide boxes, 206
  centration, 203–204
  clips, 155, 195
  labelling, 55, 205
  mailers, 206
  transport, 138, 205–206
Slides
  broken, 209–210
  cleaning, 200–201
Sliding microtomes, 60, 77, 87–88, 89, 92–93, 115, 118
Smears, 1, 2, 17, 25, 28, 142, 143, 210
Sodium ethoxide, 72
Softening fluids, 73–74, 76–77, 123–124
Spherical aberration, 196
Spray fixatives, 13, 22, 138–139, 178
Spurr's resin, 66–67
Squashes, 1, 145
Staining

automatic, 177, 179
intravital, 1, 183
procedures, 167–169
supravital, 1, 183
Stains
acidic, 160–161, 164, 174
action, 160–161
amphoteric, 160–161, 174, 177
anionic, 22, 160, 166–167, 177
bacterial, 184–186
basic, 160–161, 174, 202
cationic, 22, 160, 193
definition, 159
direct, 161, 167
fat, 22, 161, 192
free-floating, 97, 104, 119, 169, 171, 193
heating, 35, 168, 186
indirect, 161
non-ionic, 161
resin material, 172–173
ripening, 163
standardization, 175, 187–188
use, 159
Static, 24, 102–103, 124–125
Steedman's ester wax, 59
Stockwell's bleach, 78
Storing blocks, 56, 61
Stropping, 105, 109–111, 112
Strops, 109–111, 112
Subbed slides — see Gelatin-coated slides
Sulphuric acid, 19, 74, 201
Supports, non-glass, 1–2
SUSA — see Heidenhain's SUSA

Taxonomy, 3, 137
Technique, choice of, 5
Temporary mounts, 146, 183
TESPA, 198–199
Thermoplastic cements, 152–153
Tilt, 93
Tissue
cassettes, 40, 89
choppers, 96, 125, 127, 130–131
culture chambers, 146–147, 148, 183
freezing, 97–100
processors, 21, 44–45
reclamation, 64, 210–211
shrinkage, 17,18, 20, 23, 24, 27, 28, 64, 120–123, 207
storage, 23, 24, 56, 61, 104–105
swelling, 17, 18, 25, 120–123
washers, 29–30, 31
Tissues
brittle, 22, 41, 96, 124
delicate, 16, 192, 147–148
dried, 56, 210–211
embedding, 43–50, 57–62, 63–72, 99, 125, 132–133
flat, 58, 62

fluid, see Smears and Fluid mounts
friable, 26, 123, 124, 192, 198, 208
orientation, 47, 62–63, 100, 114, 149–150
refractory, 52, 77, 124, 131
softening, 72–79, 123, 124
trimming, 50–51, 99, 101, 127
Toluene, 42, 61, 193
Toluidine blue, 65, 172
Tool-edge knife, 75, 91–92, 108
Tough tissues, 23, 24, 25, 39, 43, 45, 60, 114, 131, 165, 198
Transition media, 39, 42–43, 47, 56, 66, 121, 169, 192–193
Transport, 138, 205–206
Triacetin, 165
Trichloroethane, 45
Trichrome stains, 179–183
Tüllgren funnel, 4
Tungsten carbide knife — see Tool-edge knife

UV radiation, 68, 69, 70, 71, 72, 148

Vacuum, 47, 61, 66
van Gieson, 164, 170–171
Vapour fixation, 16
Vasodilators, 15
Viability counts, 183–184
Vibratomes, 96, 125, 127, 130–131
Vice — see Chucks
Vital stains, 162, 183–184
von Orth's, 13, 26

Warming box, 156, 157
Washing tissues, 28, 29–30, 31, 75, 77, 165
Watch glass, 46, 50
Water-based mountants — see Aqueous mountants
Water-bath method, 53–54
Wax
embedding, 46–50, 76, 121, 132
embedding machines, 48
disadvantages, 63–64
melting points, 111–112, 125
stars and streaks, 47
structure, 112–113, 125
Wedge knife, 90–91, 101
Whole mounts, 1, 2, 137, 147–157, 164, 166
Woody tissues, 23, 24, 25, 27
Wright's stain, 174, 176
Wrinkles — see Folds

XAM, 194, 201
Xylene, 42, 56, 60, 76, 193

Zenker's, 13, 21, 24, 164, 187
Zenker-formol, 13, 24
see also Helly's
Ziehl-Neelsen stain, 160, 186

Lightning Source UK Ltd.
Milton Keynes UK
20 October 2009

145212UK00001B/23/A